SURVIVAL FITNESS

THE ULTIMATE FITNESS PLAN FOR ESCAPE, EVASION, AND SURVIVAL

SAM FURY

Illustrated by
DIANA MANGOBA, NEIL GERMIO, OKIANG LUHUNG, RAUL GUAJARDO, & YOPI MUHAMAD

Copyright SF Nonfiction Books © 2013

Last updated 2021 ©

www.SFNonfictionBooks.com

All Rights Reserved
No part of this document may be reproduced without written consent from the author.

WARNINGS AND DISCLAIMERS

The information in this publication is made public for reference only.

Neither the author, publisher, nor anyone else involved in the production of this publication is responsible for how the reader uses the information or the result of his/her actions.

CONTENTS

Introduction   xi

GENERAL HEALTH AND FITNESS

Nutrition	3
Life Force	8

BODY CONDITIONING

SFP Super-burpee	13
Pull-ups	23

SFP YOGA STRETCH ROUTINE

Mountain Pose	27
Standing Backbend	29
Crescent Moon	30
Standing Forward Fold	31
Table Pose	32
Threading the Needle	33
Upward Dog	34
Downward Dog	35
Low Warrior	36
Half Prayer-Twist	37
Half-Pyramid	38
Extended Dog	39
Hero Pose	40
Lion Pose	41
Downward-Facing Frog	42
Staff Pose	43
Seated Forward Bend	44
Bound Angle	45
Seated Angle	47
Side Seated Angle	48
Joyful Baby	49
Wind-Relieving Pose	50

Supine Bound Angle	51
Corpse Pose	52
Yoga Stretch Routine Quick List	53
Yoga Nidra	55

PARKOUR

Training for Reality	63

SAFETY

Safety Tap	69
Safety Rolls	71
Break-Falling	79

WARM-UPS AND CONDITIONING

Catwalk	87
Balance	89
Side Sapiens	93
Ground Kongs	95
Pull-ups	97

RUNNING AND JUMPING

Sprinting	101
Evasive Running	105
Hurdles	108
Precision Jumping	111
Crane Landing	115
Striding	117
Stride to Safety Step	119
Dive Roll	121
Parkour Runs	125
Parkour Games	126

VAULTS

Safety Vault	129
Speed Vault	132
Turn Vault	135
Reverse Safety Vault	138
Lazy Vault	140

Kong Vault	143
Reverse Vault	148

WALL TECHNIQUES

Cat Leap to Cat Hang	155
Cat to Cat	158
Tic-Tac	160
Wall Climb-up	162
Vertical Wall Run	166
Wall Pop-up	169
Corner Wall Run	171

BAR TECHNIQUES

Straight Underbar	175
Lache	178
Monkey Traverse	182
Muscle-ups	183

BOULDERING

Basic Principles	189
Holds and Grips	191
Foot Techniques	198
Mantle	202
Types of Faces	203
Crack Climbing	205

SWIMMING

TREADING WATER

Sculling	211
Eggbeater Kick (Rotary Kick)	213
Treading Water	214

SWIMMING QUICKLY

Entry and Initial Propulsion	217
Underwater Fly-Kick	225
Freestyle	229

SWIMMING LONG DISTANCES

Survival Backstroke	241
Combat Sidestroke	243

SWIMMING LONG DISTANCES UNDERWATER

Safety	251
Stage One: Dry-Land Breath-Holding	252
Stage Two: Static Underwater Breath-Holding	254
Stage Three: Static Apnea Training	255
Stage Four: Efficient Stroke	258
Stage Five: 50m Swim	260

MOUNTAIN BIKE RIDING

Basic Riding Skills	263
Basic Drills	264
Advanced Skills	268

HIKING

General Hiking Tips	275
Specific Hiking Tips	277
References	281
Author Recommendations	283
About Sam Fury	285

THANKS FOR YOUR PURCHASE

Did you know you can get FREE chapters of any SF Nonfiction Book you want?

https://offers.SFNonfictionBooks.com/Free-Chapters

You will also be among the first to know of FREE review copies, discount offers, bonus content, and more.

Go to:

https://offers.SFNonfictionBooks.com/Free-Chapters

Thanks again for your support.

INTRODUCTION

This book (Survival Fitness) is self-training in the five most useful activities for escaping danger. The idea is that if you are going to exercise, you may as well learn life-saving skills at the same time. It is the ultimate in functional fitness training.

Survival Fitness includes:

- The full version of *Daily Health and Fitness*
- The full version of *Essential Parkour*
- Bouldering
- Efficient swimming
- Mountain-bike riding
- Hiking

The point of Survival Fitness is not to be a master in all the activities. Although this is possible, it takes a lot of training, and most people will not have the time or motivation.

Instead, the aim is to increase fitness and skill to an above-average level (in comparison to the general population) in all of the activities. This will give you best overall chance of survival when you're in danger.

GENERAL HEALTH AND FITNESS

This section contains a complete body and mind health routine in four parts.

Do all four parts every day for optimal health.

1. **Nutrition.** What you put into your body matters—a lot
2. **Body Conditioning.** Two extremely efficient exercises to keep your whole body strong, including the awesome SFP Super-burpee.
3. **SFP Yoga Stretch Routine.** Stretch your whole body using this specially designed 15-minute yoga routine.
4. **Yoga Nidra.** A quick Yoga Nidra session as a form of daily meditation.

The nutrition guidelines provided here should be observed at all times. If you do the other three things back to back, they will take you less than 45 minutes. They can also be easily split up throughout the day to suit your schedule.

Be diligent in doing the above, and in under 45 minutes a day, you will be healthier in body and mind **than the majority of people on the planet!**

NUTRITION

These Survival Fitness Plan nutrition guidelines are easy to remember to stick with.

There are five major guidelines:

1. Fast for 16 hours a day.
2. Eat gut-healthy food.
3. Eat a plant-based, whole-foods diet.
4. Minimize refined sugar.
5. Minimize drug use.

16-Hour Fasting

This is intermittent fasting. There are several ways to do it, but I find this one way the best because it becomes part of your daily routine. It keeps things simple.

The stretch of time you choose depends on your lifestyle; all that matters is that it is 16 hours long. I like to fast between 8:00 p.m. and 12:00 p.m. the following day. All I'm doing is skipping breakfast.

During the fasting period, you can drink water, herbal tea, or black coffee. If you get hungry, try having a tablespoon of apple cider vinegar in a glass of water. A tablespoon of coconut oil is also good. You should consume these two things every day anyway. Both are good for your health.

Intermittent fasting has some great benefits. For example, it:

- Boosts the immune system
- Facilitates fat loss
- Improves longevity
- Lowers the risk of diabetes
- Helps you sleep better

- Slows aging
- Helps you think clearer

Eat Gut-Healthy Food

A healthy gut means a healthy mind and body. This is a scientific fact!

There are many food that are good for your guts. Kefir is one of the best, but if that's not your thing, then any fermented foods are good too. Apple cider vinegar, sauerkraut, kimchi, tempeh, miso, and pickles are all good examples.

You should also eat foods that are high in fiber, such as whole grains, beans, legumes, and whole fruits and veggies. Aim to get a good dose of high-fiber and fermented foods every day.

Plant-Based Whole Foods

What are whole foods? Here is a definition straight from Wikipedia:

"Whole foods are plant foods that are unprocessed and unrefined, or processed and refined as little as possible, before being consumed. Examples of whole foods include whole grains, tubers, legumes, fruits, vegetables."

https://en.wikipedia.org/wiki/Whole_food

As a bonus, eating a whole-foods diet will cut your food bill—by quite a lot, in some cases.

Anything made with white flour is not a whole food. This includes bread, cereals, crackers, granola bars, pasta, etc. You can still eat these things, but choose the non-white whole grain version instead. The same goes for white rice. Eat wild or brown rice instead. "Normal" potatoes are okay, but sweet potatoes are way better.

Here's a list of no white-flour foods:

https://www.livestrong.com/article/336585-list-of-no-white-flour-foods

Eat Less Refined Sugar

Refined sugar is poison, and is in many things. Here are some examples. The less of these things you eat, the healthier you'll be.

Processed food. Almost everything processed will have refined sugar in it. This covers most things that are not in the fresh-food section of the supermarket. The easiest way to know is by looking at the ingredients label.

Deep-fried foods. Most things that are deep-fried will also have refined sugar. Even if they don't, nothing deep-fried is good for you anyway.

Drinks. Drinks other than water and fresh herbal tea usually have quite a bit of sugar in them. Soft drinks are the worst. Clean water is the best drink you can have. Making it your main drink will flush your body of toxins. Aim to drink **at least** one liter every day. Herbal teas, either cold- or hot-brewed, are a good way to add a bit of flavor, as well as to get some extra benefits (such as aiding digestion and boosting your immunity).

Every morning when you wake, rinse your mouth out and then drink a couple of cups of water. It will assist rehydration from the night and stimulate your digestive system.

Minimize Drug Use

This includes alcohol, cigarettes, pharmaceuticals you don't need, and illicit drugs.

Of course, some drugs are worse than others. Smoking cigarettes, for example, is crazy. Drinking a little alcohol once in a while, not so bad.

Additional Healthy Eating Tips

Fruits. Fruits are great, but due to the large amount of fructose in them, consuming too many is bad for your teeth. Limit yourself to three servings a day.

Vegetables. You cannot eat too many vegetables. They should make up a big part of your diet. Local fruits and vegetables that are in season in your location are best.

Herbs. Not only do they make your food taste nicer, they are super healthy. Garlic, ginger, and chili are my favorites, and they are very cheap to buy and easy to grow. Garlic is crazy healthy.

Putting them in fresh salads or soups or steaming them are the best ways to prepare your vegetables. The next best is thing is to stir-fry or roast them. Stay away from deep-fried foods.

Bright or deep colors are best. Go for leafy greens, berries, red bell peppers, papaya, moringa, etc.

Wash all fruits and vegetables. Even organic fruits and vegetables can have poison sprayed on them. Ensure that you use water you would consider safe to drink.

Get a good variety. Different foods have different nutritional values. When it comes to fruit and vegetables, choose a variety of colors and types. This actually applies to all foods. Ensure you are consuming proteins, dairy, fruit, vegetables, complex carbohydrates, good fats, etc.

Proteins. Vegetarian proteins (tofu, eggs, beans, etc.) are best for health and other reasons. Failing that, go for fish (salmon is great) and lean meats (skinless chicken and lean beef are my favorites).

When you crave something sweet, go for dark chocolate. The higher the percentage of cocoa, the better. Raw honey is also great.

Benefits of Being Vegetarian

If you think you need meat for a balanced diet, you're incorrect. There are lots of replacement options, such as tofu, legumes, nuts, eggs, etc.

There are a few reasons I advocate vegetarianism:

- It's much healthier than most people realize.
- It removes the animal cruelty factor, especially with factory farming. It would be even better to go vegan.
- It saves money. In most cases, being vegetarian is cheaper than eating meat.

Here's a link to a documentary called *Mad Cowboy*. It's worth the watch:

www.youtube.com/watch?v=piZmH4gzyqs

LIFE FORCE

The life force is a non-physical essential energy that is present in all things in the universe, and the universe provides it in abundance for all.

Although the concept of the life force is rejected by modern science, the notion of it is present in most cultures, both Eastern and Western. Depending on where you are from, you may know it as chi, élan vital, gi, khi, ki, manitou, prana, ruah, qi, vitalism, etc.

In living creatures, this essential energy flows through the body. If it gets blocked, the blockage is manifested as illness and/or pain.

This means that any "sickness" you have, whether it be physical, mental, or emotional, is caused by blocked energy, and can be alleviated by releasing the blockage. It also means that sickness can be prevented by maintaining clear passages of this energy through the body. The simplest way to encourage and maintain the flow of this energy through the body is the breath.

Life Force and the Breath

Although every breath you take helps to circulate the life force throughout your body, taking full breaths is much more effective. Unfortunately, most people do not do so.

When you take the time to concentrate on proper breathing, it will promote better breathing even when you're not concentrating on it. It takes a cycle of nine breaths for the first breath to be exhaled from the body. I recommend doing four cycles of conscious breathing a day. These can be done all at once (36 breaths) or nine at a time at various times during the day.

Doing the Yoga Stretch Routine will cover 36 conscious breaths and then some. But you can do them whenever you want. The more, the better.

If you only want to do one thing a day to maintain your health, do conscious breathing.

Receiving the Breath

Get in a comfortable position. You can be lying, sitting, or standing. Completely exhale your whole breath. This is the effortful part.

Now just allow the inhale to come in naturally through your nose. There is no need to actively breathe in deeply. Just receive it. Over time, you'll notice that your breaths naturally get deeper.

As you breathe in and out it, may help to imagine the flow of energy carried by your breath. It comes up your back as you inhale, and down your front as you exhale.

Inhale all the goodness of a new positive energy, and exhale all the stale and negative.

Three-Part Breath

This is the breath you should do when actively practicing yoga, but when first learning it, you'll probably just want to do it from a sitting or lying position.

Breathe in long and deep through your nose. First, feel it enter your lower belly, then your lower chest/rib cage, and finally your lower throat/ the top of your sternum. Feel the clear, positive energies of happiness and love come up from your toes to your head.

When you are ready, exhale fully through your nose, feeling the breath leave in the opposite order from the one it came in— that is, first from your sternum, then from your chest, and finally from your belly. Release all negative energy and tension out of your body, from your head to your toes. Continue to breathe in and out like this, smoothly and continuously.

When you first start to practice this type of breathing, it may help to put your hands on each of the three areas (belly, chest, and sternum) as you do it. You can also try just breathing into each area on its own.

BODY CONDITIONING

This section describes two exercises designed to keep your physical body strong in the most efficient way.

5 SFP super-burpees is the bare minimum of daily exercise.

The ideal daily conditioning routine is:

- 10 SFP super-burpees
- 10 pull-ups

SFP SUPER-BURPEE

The Survival Fitness Plan (SFP) super-burpee is an extremely efficient exercise that acts as a warm-up, light stretch, and full-body muscle conditioning workout all in one.

When several super-burpees are done properly and in succession, they also serve to fill the body with life force, as well as to give a cardiovascular workout. Furthermore, the exercise has been tweaked over time to give additional benefits in relation to SFP fight and flight activities such as parkour and self-defense.

Here is a list of the main benefits gained from the SFP super-burpee:

- Balance
- Cardiovascular workout
- Circulation of life force
- Coordination
- Explosiveness
- Improved bodily function (digestion, respiration, etc.)
- Flexibility
- Muscle conditioning
- Hang time (the ability to stay airborne)
- Striking strength and speed
- Warm-up

I highly recommended doing **at least** five SFP super-burpees every morning to ready your body for the day. One SFP super-burpee takes less than 10 seconds.

Even if you only have one minute to spare for exercise, you have time to do SFP super-burpees!

I also recommend doing SFP super-burpees as a general warm-up before any vigorous exercise, such as SFP Fight and Flight training.

The SFP super-burpee is made up of five separate exercises, each of which has been specifically chosen and tweaked to provide the most benefit in relation to the Survival Fitness Plan.

Jumping squats: Jumping squats develop leg strength, core strength, explosiveness, soft landing skills, jumping ability, and hang-time.

Finger-tip push-ups: Finger-tip push-ups increase finger strength and grip, increase striking power, and improve all-over body conditioning.

Clapping push-ups: These are great for increasing striking power and all-over body conditioning. The clapping part really improves explosiveness, which is awesome for speed and power. The push-up also condition your hands for the palm-heel strike which is preferred over a fist in SFP Self-Defense training.

Hindu Push-ups: Hindu push-ups use the downward dog and the upward dog (yoga poses) which are beneficial for your:

- Brain (stimulates)
- Breathing (chest)
- Concentration
- Eyesight
- Hearing
- Kidneys
- Memory
- Nervous system
- Spine
- Whole-body strengthening

Brazilians: Brazilians mainly contribute to cardiovascular workout and hip flexibility, but they also increase core strength and work the lower abdominals.

If you are unable to do a full SFP super-burpee, you can build yourself up to them by doing each individual exercise separately.

Once you can do each 10 repetitions of each individual exercise, you should be strong enough to put them together into an SFP super-burpee.

The first SFP super-burpee you do for the day (or when warming up for exercise) must be done slowly and with much purpose.

If you try to do fast super-burpees straight away, your chances of injury will greatly increase. Doing the first one very well will warm up and stretch your body. After that, you can gradually increase speed with the second and third repetitions until you are going full-speed for as many reps as you can handle.

Note: If you have any injuries, please leave out any part of the SFP super-burpee that may aggravate them.

The following is a detailed explanation of how to do a full SFP super-burpee as if it's the first one.

Jumping Squat

Stand straight, with your feet shoulder-width apart.

As you breathe in, squat down as low as you can. Keep your back straight and come up on your toes as you squat down. Put your arms out to your front. This will help you keep your back straight.

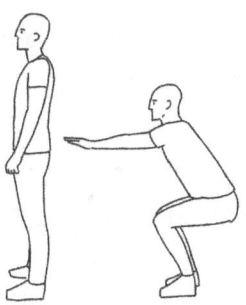

Spring up as you exhale, and jump as high as you can. Tuck your legs up as high as possible on the outside of your elbows. Try to keep your back straight. This is actually a box jump.

Land as softly as you can, and adopt a crouching squat position.

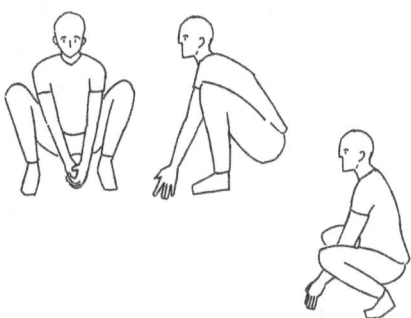

Note: If you can't do a jumping squat, you can build up to one by doing regular squats first. Just do as explained above, but without the jump.

Finger-tip push-up

From the squat position, as you inhale, place your fingertips firmly on the ground next to your feet and shoot both your legs behind you, so you're in the standard up position for a push-up, with the exception of being on your fingertips.

Ensure that your elbows are as close to your torso as possible, and that they are facing back towards your feet. This is so you target the muscles used for striking.

Grip the floor with your fingers, as if you're trying to rip a chunk out of the ground. Keep this grip throughout the push-up.

As you inhale, lower your chest until your arms are at a 90° angle at the elbow.

Push back up as fast as possible to the up position.

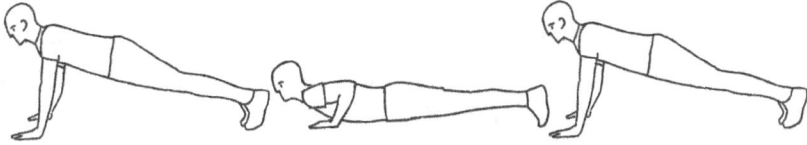

Clapping Push-up

Lower your chest again as you inhale.

This time, as you exhale, push up hard enough for you to be able to get your hands off the ground and clap.

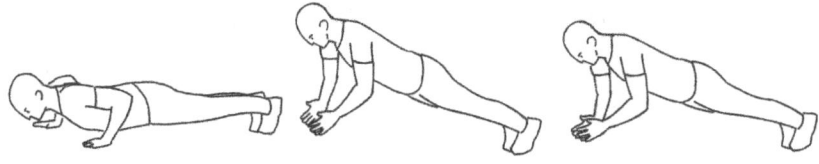

Aim to land on the palms of your hands as softly as possible and then return to the up position of the push-up.

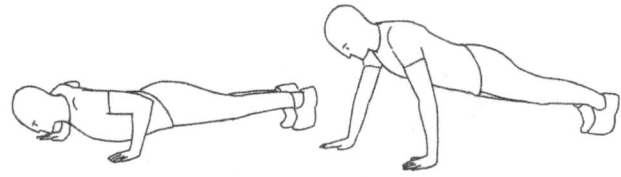

Note: If you can't do either of these push-ups, work your way up to them with normal push-ups. Next, do finger-tip pushups, and then clapping pushups.

If you can't yet do a normal push-up, work your way up to it first by just lying on your stomach and pushing up. Push on the ground for 10 seconds, and then rest. This is one rep. Do three sets of three reps every day. Eventually you'll be able to do a push-up. Once you can do 10 normal push-ups, try for fingertip push-ups.

It will help to do finger-strengthening exercises as well. A simple and very effective one is to place your fingertips together and push them against each other for as long as you can. Do it every day until you are able to do fingertip push-ups.

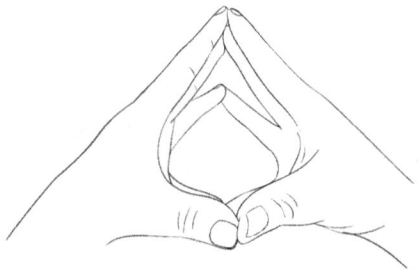

Hindu Push-up

From the up position of the push-up, breathe in and go into downward dog. If this is your first SFP super-burpee, spend a couple of breaths here to stretch your body. Go up on each foot to stretch your legs and really extend your upper body.

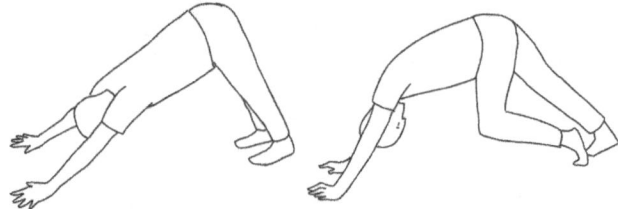

As you breathe out, sweep down in a circular arc motion into upward dog.

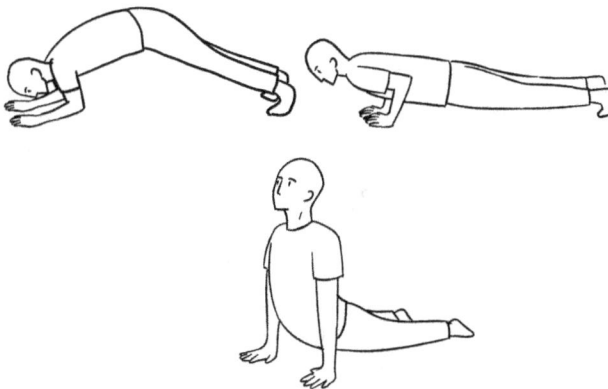

Again, if this is your first SFP super-burpee, spend a couple of breaths here to stretch your body.

Really arch your back and look high above. Move your neck from side to side and stretch out your arms, back, and upper thighs. When you're ready, inhale and return to the up position of the push-up.

Brazilians

As you exhale, bring your right knee to your left elbow and then back. Then bring your left knee to your right elbow. This is one rep of a Brazilian.

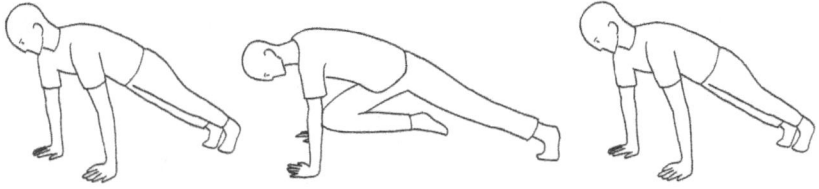

Jump back into a squat and then stand up straight.

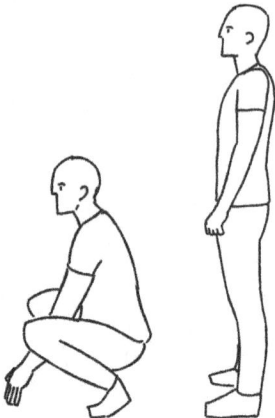

This completes one repetition of an SFP super-burpee.

General Health and Fitness

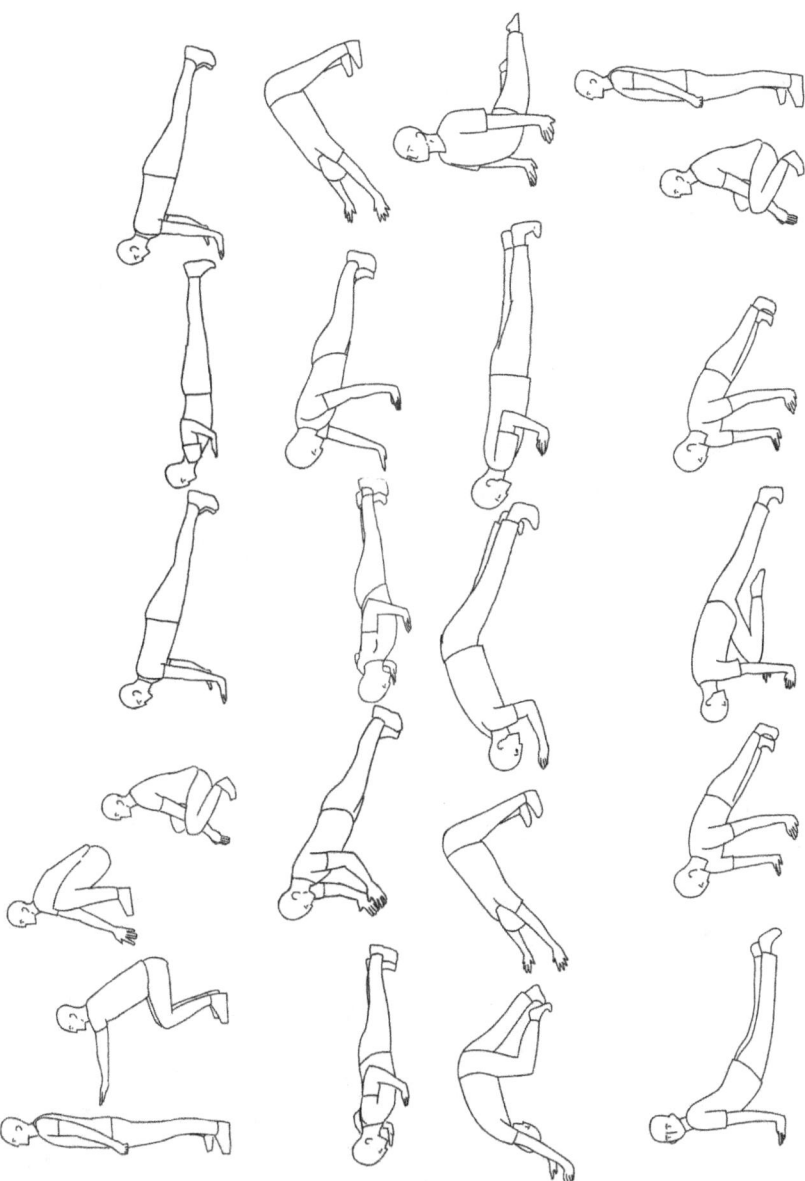

A complete SFP super-burpee

Related Chapters:

- Life Force
- Upward Dog
- Downward Dog

PULL-UPS

Being able to pull yourself up is an extremely useful skill, and the best way to condition yourself to do so is with the classic pull-up.

The pull-up is an especially useful exercise for the Survival Fitness Plan. It helps you build strength for parkour wall-climbs and, eventually, muscle-ups.

You can find a description of how to do pull-ups in the Parkour section of this book.

Related Chapters:

- Pull-ups

SFP YOGA STRETCH ROUTINE

The Survival Fitness Plan (SFP) yoga cool-down is a whole body stretch which also gives the many other benefits of yoga. Balance, a calm mind, coordination, core strength, development of chi, flexibility, etc.

This yoga cool-down is approximately 15 minutes long if you stay in each pose for two to three breaths. The longer you stay in each pose for, the more beneficial it is, so go longer than 15 minutes if you want.

Whilst doing this routine it is important to move slowly and use conscious breathing.

Although all the poses used in this book are considered basic ones, you may find some of them challenging when you're first starting.

Adjust them to your comfort level and work your way up. Hold each pose to the point where you can feel a good stretch, but not pain.

You will probably notice your breath shorten if you try to force your body too much. When this happens, just back off a little and refocus on your breathing. If you do find yourself in a painful position, back out of it slowly to avoid injury.

Note: If you are planning to do more physical exercise as part of this routine, do it after conditioning and before this yoga stretch routine.

The information in this section is from the book *Curing Yoga* by Aventuras De Viaje.

www.SFNonfictionBooks.com/Curing-Yoga

MOUNTAIN POSE

Avoid this if you have a shoulder injury.

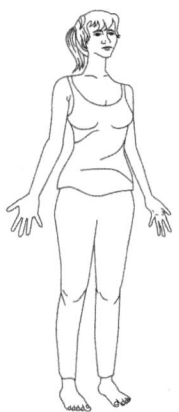

Stand with your feet parallel and either together or hip-width apart.

Spread your toes wide and balance your weight evenly and centrally over each foot.

Pull up your kneecaps and tense your thighs. Keep your legs straight, but do not lock your knees. Ensure your hips are directly over your ankles.

As you inhale, lengthen your spine so that the crown of your head goes straight up towards the sky.

When you exhale, drop your shoulders and stretch your fingertips towards the ground, whilst still extending your head upwards. At the same time, gently push your chest straight ahead.

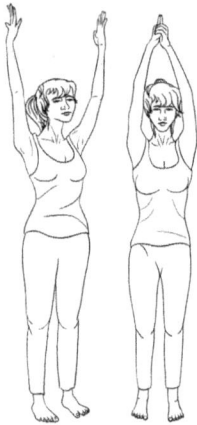

While continuing to stretch your fingertips, inhale and bring your arms up above your head to reach for the sky, palms facing each other.

As you exhale, relax your shoulders, but continue to stretch your crown and fingers towards the sky. An alternative position is to interlace your fingers with your index fingers pointing up.

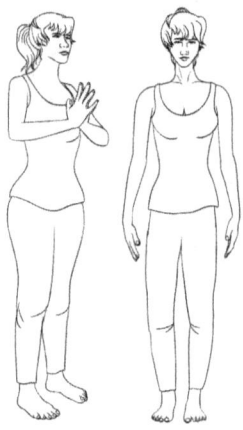

When you're ready, exhale and bring your palms together in front of your chest in a prayer position. Take a breath, and allow your hands to drop to your sides on the exhale.

STANDING BACKBEND

Avoid this if you have a back, hip, and/or neck injury.

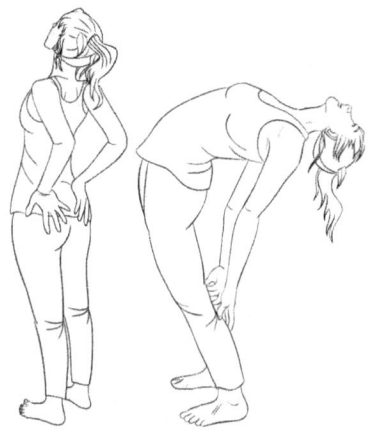

Stand with your feet parallel and hip-width apart.

As you breathe in, place the palms of your hands on your lower back (sacrum) with your fingers pointing to the ground.

Squeeze your buttocks and thighs tightly together, pull up your kneecaps, and press into your feet.

Exhale and press your hips forward as you arch your back.

You can either look straight ahead or allow your head to drop all the way back.

Increase the stretch by walking your hands down the back of your legs.

When you're ready, slowly come back to a standing position with your hands by your sides.

CRESCENT MOON

Avoid this if you have a back, hip, and/or shoulder injury.

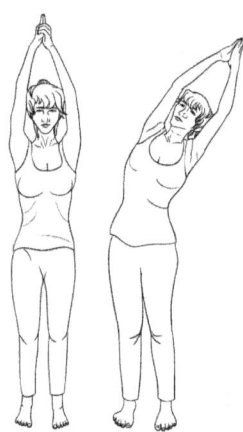

Stand with your feet parallel and either together or hip-width apart.

While inhaling, join your hands together above your head with your fingers interlaced and your index fingers pointing to the sky.

As you exhale, push your left hip out to the side and arch to your left. Keep your body strong and lengthened.

Inhale as you return to the position, with your fingers interlaced and your index fingers pointing to the sky. Repeat it on your other side.

STANDING FORWARD FOLD

Avoid this if you have a back, hip, leg, and/or shoulder injury.

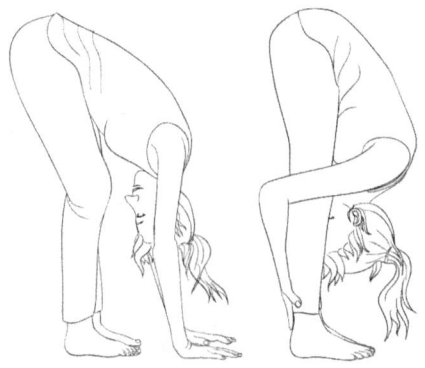

Stand with your feet parallel and either together or hip-width apart.

Exhale and bring your head to your knees, with your palms flat on the floor.

Stretch your spine by pulling your head down while pushing your hips up. Bend your knees if you need to, but aim to be able to do it with straight legs. Press your belly into your thighs when inhaling.

For a deeper stretch, hold the back of your calves and pull your head closer to your legs.

TABLE POSE

Avoid this if you have a knee and/or wrist injury.

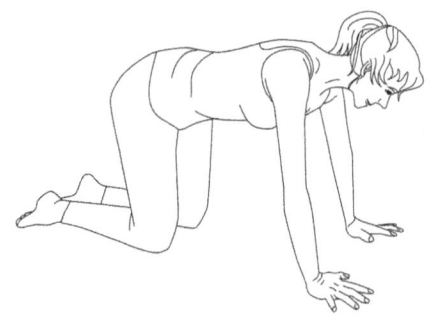

As you inhale, place your hands and knees on the floor, with your palms directly underneath your shoulders and fingers facing forward.

Ensure your knees are shoulder-width apart and your feet are directly behind them, with the tops of your feet and toes on the floor.

Look at the ground between your hands and press down into your palms.

Have your back flat and exhale while lengthening your spine by pressing the crown of your head forward and your tailbone back.

THREADING THE NEEDLE

Avoid this if you have a knee, neck, and/or shoulder injury.

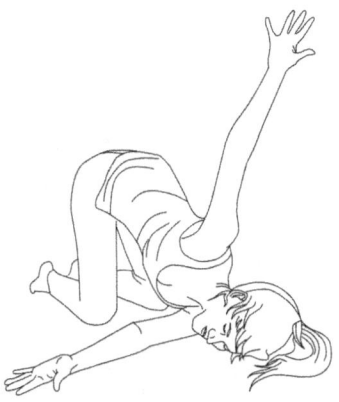

Place your hands and knees on the floor, with your palms directly underneath your shoulders and fingers facing forward. Your knees are shoulder-width apart and your feet are directly behind them. Have your back flat.

As you exhale, slide your right hand between your left knee and left hand until your right shoulder and the side of your head are resting on the floor.

Inhale and reach towards the sky with your left hand. Find where you get the deepest stretch and stay there, reaching out with your fingers.

When you're ready, exhale as you bring your hand back to the floor and then inhale to readopt your starting position.

Repeat on your left side.

UPWARD DOG

Avoid if you have an arm, back, hip, and/or shoulder injury, have had recent abdominal surgery, and/or are pregnant.

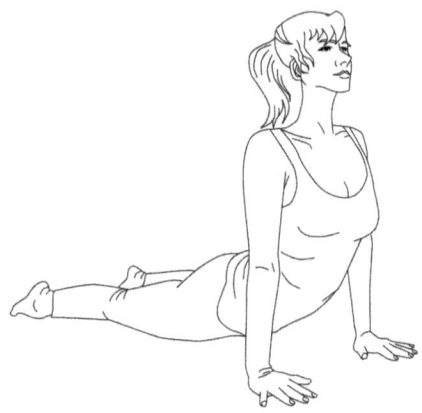

Place your hands and knees on the floor, with your palms directly underneath your shoulders and fingers facing forward. Your knees are shoulder-width apart and your feet are directly behind them. Have your back flat.

Drop your hips forward towards the ground as you press your palms down into the floor.

Press your chest forward as you drop your shoulders down and back.

Push the crown of your head towards the ceiling.

As you inhale, press the tops of your feet into the ground to lift your legs off the floor. Only the tops of your feet and your hands should touch the ground. Press all of your toenails firmly into the floor.

DOWNWARD DOG

Avoid this if you have an arm, back, hip, and/or shoulder injury, and/or unmediated high blood pressure.

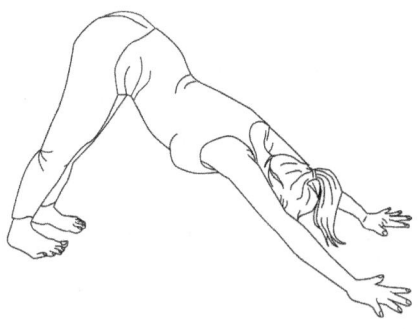

Place your hands and knees on the floor, with your palms directly underneath your shoulders and fingers facing forward. Your knees are shoulder-width apart and your feet are directly behind them. Have your back flat.

As you inhale, tuck in your toes so you are on the balls of your feet. Keep your palms shoulder width apart and spread your fingers apart, with your middle fingers facing forward.

Press into your hands and lift your hips towards the sky.

Push your hips up and back. Your chest should move towards your thighs. Keep your arms straight, but don't lock your elbows.

Keep your spine straight as you lift up through your tailbone.

Stretch the backs of your legs by pressing your heels to the floor. Keep your back flat. Your legs should be straight (knees not locked) or with a small bend at the knees.

Let your head dangle freely.

LOW WARRIOR
Avoid this if you have an ankle, arm, hip, and/or shoulder injury.

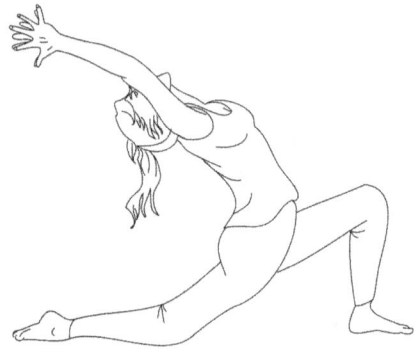

Place your hands and knees on the floor, with your palms directly underneath your shoulders and fingers facing forward. Your knees are shoulder-width apart and your feet are directly behind them. Have your back flat.

Step your right foot forward, placing it in between your hands. Your knee should be directly over your ankle.

Ensure your left knee and left and right feet are firmly on the ground, and then place your hands on your right knee.

Straighten your arms and bring your torso back. Do not lock your elbows.

Relax your shoulders and stick your chest out by bringing your shoulder blades towards each other.

As you inhale, raise your arms over your head with your palms facing each other and arch your back as you look up to the sky. If this is difficult, then you can keep your hands on your bent knee.

When you're ready, exhale as you bring your palms back to the floor on either side of your right foot.

HALF PRAYER-TWIST

Avoid this if you have a back, hip, knee, and/or shoulder injury.

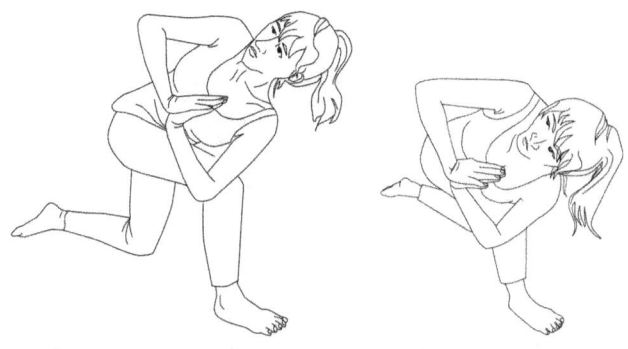

Adopt a low lunge position with your right foot forward and your left lower leg flat on the ground. Place your palms on the floor, one on each side of your front foot.

As you inhale, bring your torso up and place your hands together in a prayer position.

Place your left elbow to the outside of your right knee and use your arms to press your left shoulder up and back. Feel it twist your upper back.

Ensure your palms remain in the center of your chest with your fingers pointing towards your throat.

You can either look straight ahead or up towards the sky.

When you're ready, exhale as you bring your palms back to the floor, one on each side of your left foot.

HALF-PYRAMID

Avoid this if you have a knee and/or leg injury.

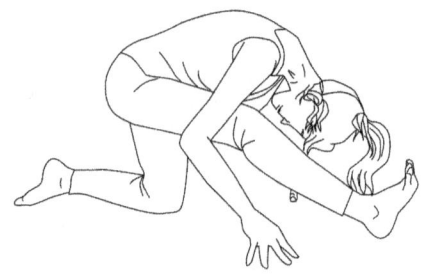

Adopt a low lunge position with your right foot forward and your left lower leg flat on the ground.

While exhaling, straighten your right leg as you press your hips back towards your left heel.

Round your spine and lift your toes to the sky as you push your forehead into your right knee. Walk your hands back towards you to support your torso. Relax your elbows, face, neck, and shoulders.

When you're ready, inhale and bend your right knee back over your ankle, and then exhale and bring your right knee back next to your left one.

EXTENDED DOG

Avoid this if you have an arm, back, knee, and/or shoulder injury.

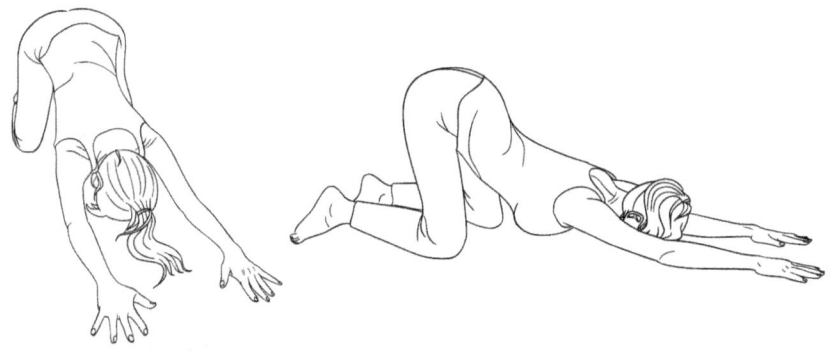

Place your hands and knees on the floor, with your palms directly underneath your shoulders and fingers facing forward. Your knees are shoulder-width apart and your feet are directly behind them. Have your back flat.

As you inhale, push your tailbone towards the sky then exhale and lower your forehead to the floor by sliding your hands forward. Ensure you keep your hips lifted over your knees.

Arch the middle of your back by allowing your chest to sink towards the floor.

Deepen the stretch by straightening your arms, lifting your elbows off the floor, and bringing your hips back. Try not to let your hands slide while you do this.

Place your chin on the ground to stretch your neck.

When you're ready, inhale and return to your starting position.

HERO POSE
Avoid this if you have a knee injury.

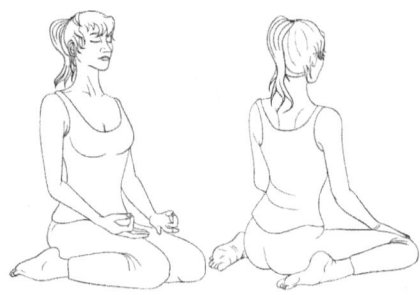

Kneel on the ground with your knees together and your feet hip-width apart. Sit with your bum on the ground and your heels on the outside of your hips. If this is too difficult, you can sit on your heels.

Place your hands on your knees. Your palms can face up or down.

Lengthen your torso by reaching the crown of your head to the sky.

Push your lower legs into the ground, drop your shoulders, and press your chest forward.

Relax your belly, face, jaw, and tongue.

Hero pose is an excellent pose for rest and/or meditation.

LION POSE

Avoid this if you have a face, knee, neck, and/or tongue injury.

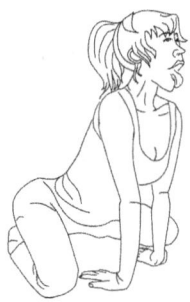

Kneel on the ground with your knees together and your feet hip-width apart. Sit with your bum on the ground and your heels on the outside of your hips.

Bring your feet together and spread your knees as wide as you comfortably can.

Sit on your heels.

Inhale and lengthen your spine by stretching the crown of your head towards the sky.

Bring your palms to the floor in between your knees, with your fingers facing your body.

Arch your spine, stick your tongue out, and exhale ferociously via your mouth.

Repeat this a few times.

DOWNWARD-FACING FROG

Avoid this if you have a knee, hip, and/or leg injury.

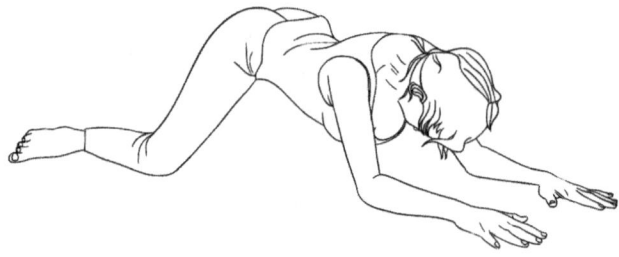

Kneel on the ground with your knees together and your feet hip-width apart. Sit with your bum on the ground and your heels on the outside of your hips.

Spread your knees as wide as you comfortably can and align your feet so that they are directly behind them—that is, with your right foot behind your right knee and your left foot behind your left knee.

Turn your feet outwards so your toes are facing away from your body.

Place your elbows, forearms, and palms flat on the floor.

Exhale as you push your hips back.

STAFF POSE

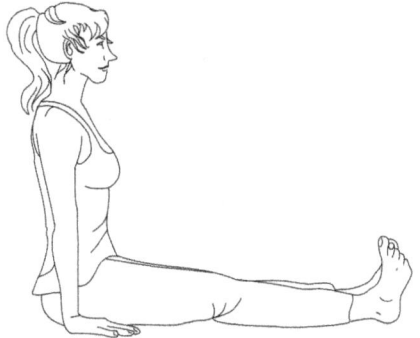

Start in a seated position with your legs extended straight out in front of you. Place your hands beside your hips with your fingers pointed forward.

Lengthen your spine by pressing your hip bones down while pushing the crown of your head towards the sky. Use your arms for support as you push your chest forward and lower your shoulders.

Pull your toes towards your head as you push your heels away from you.

SEATED FORWARD BEND
Avoid this if you have an ankle, arm, hip, and/or shoulder injury.

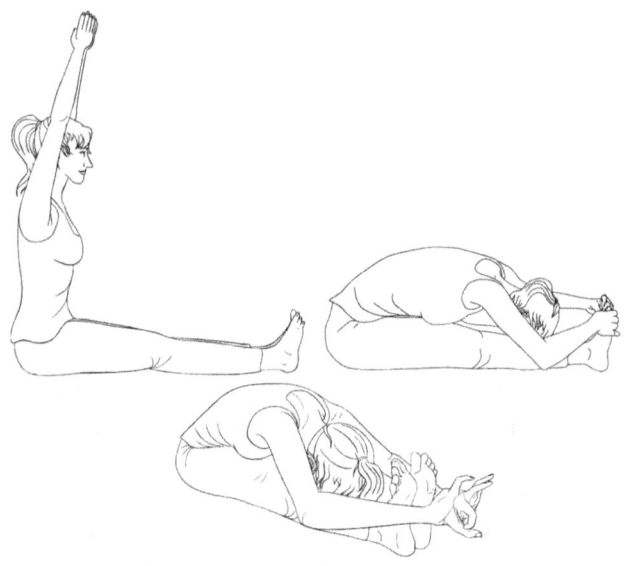

Start in a seated position with your legs extended straight out in front of you. Inhale and raise your arms up to the sky, with your palms facing each other. Lengthen your torso through your fingers and the crown of your head.

As you exhale, bend at the hips, lowering your upper body to your legs. Grab your ankles, feet, or toes.

Push out through your heels as you pull your toes back towards you.

You can use your arms to pull yourself closer to your legs. If you have more flexibility, reach your hands in front of your feet. If you're having difficulties, bend your knees enough so that you can reach your feet and place your head on your knees.

When you're ready, slowly roll up your spine back into the seated position.

BOUND ANGLE
Avoid this if you have a hip and/or knee injury.

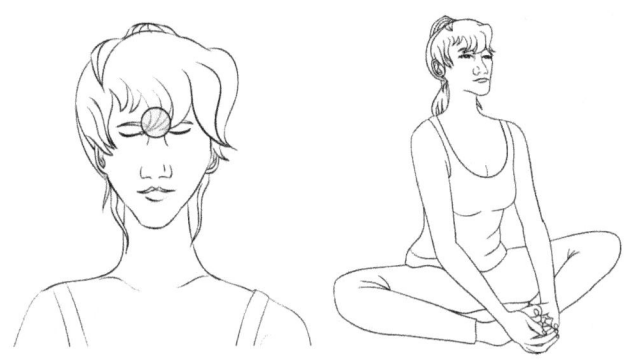

Start in a seated position with your legs extended straight out in front of you.

Bend your legs to bring the bottoms of your feet together. Your knees should bend outwards. Hold onto your toes by lacing your fingers around them.

As you inhale, stretch the crown of your head up towards the sky while pushing your hips down.

Push your chest forward and relax your shoulders down.

Close your eyes and look to your third eye (behind the middle of your forehead). As you exhale, push your knees to the ground and gently pull your torso forward.

Ensure you're keeping your chest open and your back flat.

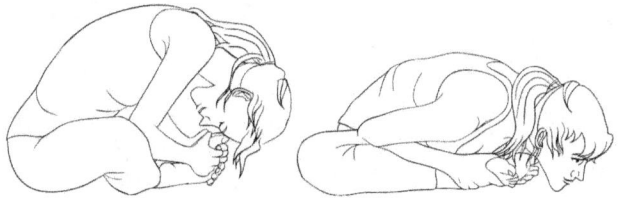

For a deeper stretch, pull your forehead or chest towards your feet. When you're ready, return to staff pose.

Related Chapters:

- Staff Pose

SEATED ANGLE

Avoid this if you have an arm, hip, knee, and/or shoulder injury.

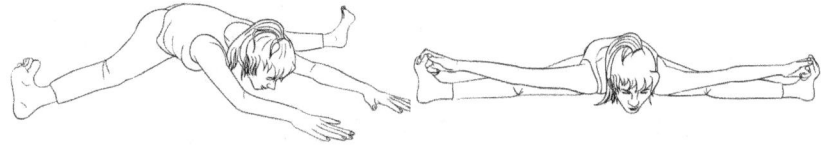

Start in a seated position with your legs extended straight out in front of you.

As you inhale, spread your legs out as wide as comfortable.

Ensure your knees and toes are pointing up and reach through your fingers up to the sky.

Exhale as you lower your palms to the floor.

Deepen the stretch by walking your hands forward. Stay focused on keeping your spine long. You could also hold your big toes and use them to help pull your torso down.

When you're ready, inhale and slowly walk your hands in as you roll back your spine until you finish with a straight back.

SIDE SEATED ANGLE
Avoid if you have a hip, leg, and/or lower back injury.

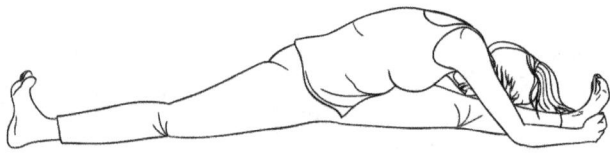

Start in a seated position with your legs spread your legs out as wide as comfortable.

Turn to face your right foot by twisting at your waist.

Walk your hands towards your right foot as you exhale. Try to reach your forehead to your knee and hold your right ankle or foot if you are able.

Relax your shoulders and neck and then increase the stretch by pressing your heel out while pulling your toes back towards yourself.

When you're ready, return to center with your back straight and then do the same thing on your left side.

JOYFUL BABY

Avoid this if you have a leg, neck, and/or shoulder injury.

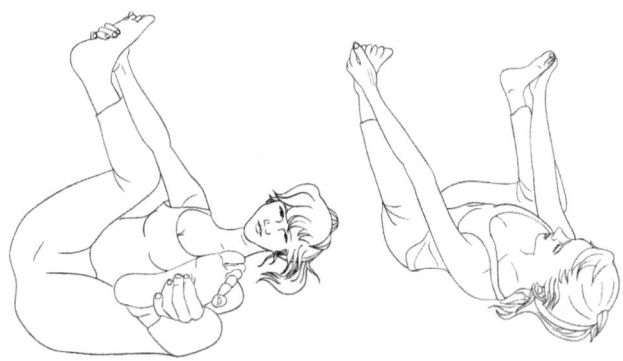

Lie flat on your back on the floor.

As you inhale, bring your knees to your chest.

Weave your arms through the inside of your knees and hold onto the pinkie-toe sides of your feet with your hands.

Keep your head on the ground and tuck your chin to your chest.

Push your heels up to the sky as you pull back with your arms. At the same time, press the back of your neck, shoulders, sacrum, and tailbone to the floor.

Open your legs wider for a deeper hip stretch.

When you're ready, exhale and slowly roll your spine back to the ground until you're lying flat again.

WIND-RELIEVING POSE

Avoid this if you have a hernia and/or have had recent abdominal surgery.

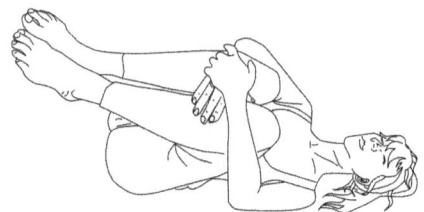

Lie flat on your back on the floor.

As you inhale, bring both knees up to your chest.

Hug your knees and hold onto the elbows, forearms, fingers, or wrists of your opposite arm (that is, hold your right arm with your left hand, and vice versa).

Keep your head on the floor while tucking your chin to your chest.

Pull your knees to your chest as you press the back of your neck, shoulders, sacrum, and tailbone to the floor. Relax your feet, hips, and legs.

Inhale deeply into your belly and press it against your thighs as you do so.

When you're ready, exhale and relax all your limbs to the ground so you are lying flat again.

SUPINE BOUND ANGLE
Avoid this if you have a hip and/or shoulder injury.

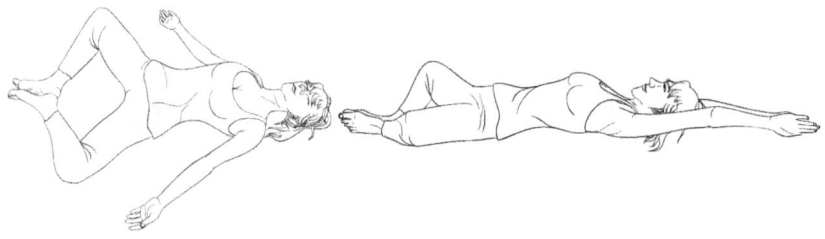

Lie flat on your back on the floor. Bend your legs to bring the bottoms of your feet together.

Your knees should face out just like in bound angle, but lying down. Allow your knees to drop to the ground.

You can rest your hands on your thighs to "encourage" them, but don't push down.

As you inhale, slide your arms on the ground over your head until your palms are together. Cross your thumbs.

When you're ready, exhale as you return to a lying position.

Related Chapters:

- Bound Angle

CORPSE POSE

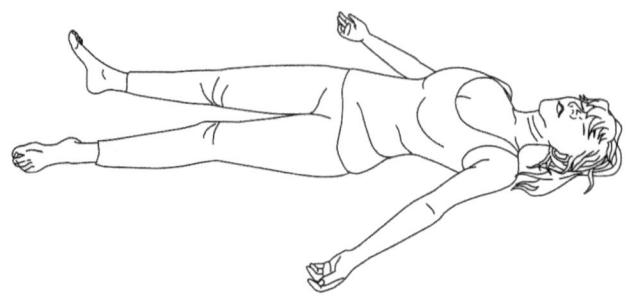

Lie flat on your back on the floor. You can place a pillow under your head if you want.

Keep your head straight; don't let it fall to the side.

Draw your shoulder blades down and open your chest towards your chin.

Have your arms at a comfortable distance from your body, with your palms facing up. Completely relax your arms and fingers.

Lift and extend your buttocks to your heels so that your whole sacrum rests on the floor.

Keep your abdomen soft and relaxed.

Slowly stretch your legs out straight, one at the time. Allow them to roll out to the side from the hips to the feet. Check that your body is in a straight line and you are resting evenly on the left and right sides.

Once you're comfortable, stay perfectly still and quiet and be aware of your body relaxing deeper into the floor. Allow your eyes to rest completely so they sink deeper towards the back of the skull. Relax your whole face and body. Be aware of your breath, quiet and soft.

Yoga Cool-Down and Stretch Routine Quick-List

Transitional poses are those with *asterisks.*

1. Mountain
2. Standing backbend
3. Crescent moon
4. Standing forward fold
5. Table
6. Threading the needle left
7. *Table*
8. Threading the needle right
9. *Table*
10. Upward dog
11. Downward dog
12. *Table*
13. Low warrior left
14. Half prayer twist left
15. Half pyramid left
16. *Table*
17. Low warrior right
18. Half prayer twist right
19. Half pyramid right
20. *Table*
21. Extended dog
22. *Table*
23. Hero
24. Lion
25. Downward frog
26. Staff
27. Seated forward bend
28. *Staff*
29. Bound angle
30. *Staff*
31. Seated angle
32. Side seated angle left
33. *Seated angle*
34. Side seated angle right
35. *Seated angle*
36. *Staff*
37. Joyful baby
38. Wind relieving
39. Supine bound angle
40. Corpse

The longer you stay in each pose, the more beneficial it is, so go longer than 15 minutes if you want.

Other than the first time they appear, table pose, staff pose, and seated angle are transitional poses (marked with *asterisks). When doing a 15-minute routine, only stay in them for a few seconds.

Related Chapters:

- Table Pose
- Staff Pose
- Seated Angle

YOGA NIDRA

Yoga Nidra is a form of guided meditation that has many health benefits. You can guide yourself, but the easiest way to do it is to listen to a Yoga Nidra practice and do what the instructor says.

The Survival Fitness Plan in to do **at least** ten minutes of Yoga Nidra immediately following the yoga cool-down.

Yoga Nidra is used in the Survival Fitness Plan because it is guided meditation, which makes it relatively easy to do, especially for beginners. If you use other forms of mediation that you enjoy, then feel free to stick to them. The main thing is that you do some sort meditation.

For best results, find a place where your body can be comfortable and you can practice undisturbed. It shouldn't be too hot or cold. Put on some soothing background music if you want.

It is best not to do Yoga Nidra in bed, because you'll be more likely to fall asleep. A yoga mat on the floor is ideal.

Yoga Nidra is a conscious practice.

Note: Ten minutes is a very short time to do Yoga Nidra. If you can spare the extra time, you can download some really good Yoga Nidra practices for free at:

YogaNidraNetwork.org/downloads.

Lie in Corpse Pose

Lie in corpse pose, as previously explained.

Corpse pose, a.k.a. shavasana, is a yoga pose used at the end of almost every yoga practice. Going straight from your yoga practice to Yoga Nidra is ideal and is (in my opinion) most likely the intention of the ones who created it.

Yoga Nidra can also be done from a sitting position if lying down is inappropriate.

Close your eyes.

Notice Your Breath

Notice your breathing. Feel your lungs filling with air, your stomach expanding, and then deflating.

Imagine a light around your body expanding and contracting as you breathe in and out. Feel the energy coursing through your body.

Use Your Senses

Notice each of your senses individually.

What sounds do you hear? Near, far, inside, outside.

What smells can you smell? Take small sniffs, like a dog does.

Taste the air.

Feel your body supported on the floor. Which parts of your body are touching?

What can you see with your eyes closed? Does the light make shapes on your eyelids?

Repeat Your Mantra

Your mantra is a short sentence stating your intentions. It's kind of like an affirmation. It may be an overall statement of health, relaxation, etc., or it may be a visualization of something you want to achieve.

Whatever it is, repeat it mentally three times. Try to feel how you would feel if the visualization was realized.

One I use often is "My entire being is completely relaxed and at one with the universe."

Scan Your Body

This is where you consciously relax each part of your body.

Mentally go through your body. Bring your attention to and relax each part. You can be very detailed about this, or just do large areas. I start from the top of my head and work my way down. Sometimes I even do internal organs.

After you have relaxed smaller body parts, relax whole sections. For example, relax your shoulder, upper arm, bicep, elbow, forearm, hand, fingers, and then your whole arm. At the end, relax your whole body as one.

Awaken the Body

The last step is to slowly deepen your breath and start to move your fingers and toes, then your hands and feet.

In your own time, stretch your body out in whatever way feels right. Open your eyes when you're ready.

When you're done stretching, gently hug your knees (wind-relieving pose). Fall to your right side and then gently sit up. Take a moment to reflect on the practice, and then go about your day.

Related Chapters:

- Wind-Relieving Pose
- Corpse Pose

PARKOUR

Parkour is one of the most useful ways to get out of immediate danger when on land.

This training manual focuses on essential parkour movements. By "essential," I mean those movements and techniques which, with basic training, would be relatively safe to use without pre-planning—if you were running away from someone in an unfamiliar area, for example.

Why Learn Parkour?

The main reason to learn parkour is the same one for which it was invented: to develop the ability to get from one point to another as efficiently as possible. There are also other benefits, such as:

- It's a fun and challenging way to keep fit. It's exercising without feeling like you're exercising. You just learn the skills; physical fitness is a welcome byproduct.

- It's a good way to socialize with other parkour enthusiasts. Or if you prefer to be a loner, parkour can be practiced solo.
- It lets you see the world around you in a new light. Once you start to learn parkour, you will no longer look at buildings, stairs, rails, or any other structure in the same way again.
- It helps you overcome fear. Many parkour movements, like jumping gaps, can be daunting, but you'll be able to draw on the confidence you gain from succeeding at them in other areas of your life.
- It increases your imagination. Figuring out different ways to get from point to point using parkour skills is good for your creativity.

Progression

Proper progression in parkour is useful for breaking through fear as well as for safety.

Conquer small milestones and gradually increase to bigger goals. After you successfully complete something once, it will get easier. But don't get too cocky. That's how injuries occur.

The techniques in this book are given in a progression according to the type of movement (landing, vault, wall, etc.), but that doesn't mean you need to learn all (or any) of one type of movement before starting to train in another. Almost any type of movement can be practiced at your discretion.

There is one exception: **Proper landing techniques, specifically the safety tap and safety rolling, should be learned first** to prevent injury.

Techniques are presented using the method taught in the Survival Fitness Plan, but there are many ways to learn the same thing. If something doesn't work for you, try it a different way. Adopt the philosophy of using what is good for you and discarding what is not.

Although parkour can be practiced solo, for most people, having a training partner helps with progression, since you will learn from and motivate each other. It's also good for safety.

TRAINING FOR REALITY

Parkour is a great skill to have if you need to run away from an enemy, but training is not the same as having to use it in real life.

Here are some things you can do to prepare yourself in case you need to use parkour in a real-life scenario.

Awareness

Constantly be aware of your surroundings. Use your peripheral vision and formulate a plan of escape whenever you enter a new situation (notice where the exits are, how you would overcome obstacles, etc.).

A side effect of this is that your being aware is obvious. People (would-be attackers) notice that you are, which makes you less of a target.

Outdoors

Train in all terrains, in all types of weather, and in all different types of light.

There are some exceptions. For example, I would not attempt some of the parkour movements on slippery surfaces.

If something is too dangerous to do during training, then it's also too dangerous to do in real life. Remember this if you ever have to make the decision about what to do.

It's also important to vary your training grounds. Training in the same place all the time will limit your imagination, and different situations will require different approaches.

Parkour and Self-Defense

It is highly recommended to combine your parkour training with self-defense. They complement each other very well. For example, the tic-tac can be integrated with a side kick.

Learn more about self-defense training at:

www.SurvivalFitnessPlan.com/Self-Defense-Tutorials

Training on Both Sides

In reality, you should favor the strong side of your body when performing actions. When training, do so on both sides so if you cannot use your strong side (due to an injury, for instance) your weaker side will still be pretty good.

What You Carry

If you habitually carry a bag and are not willing to leave it behind when threatened, then you should train with it on. The tighter the bag fits to your body, the less it will move around when training.

What You Wear

If what you wear in training is not the same thing you wear most of the time, then you won't know if you can execute parkour moves in everyday life. For example, how often do you go out with your climbing shoes on and chalk in your back pocket? If the answer is always, then feel free to use climbing shoes and chalk when training using the Survival Fitness Plan.

> *Q. So I should train in my suit and tie or skirt and high heels?*
> *A. Yes and no.*

Training in clothing that is impractical for physical exercise will hinder your progress, but you should do it at least once in a while so you know what it's like to do parkour in that type of clothing.

You may also want to consider changing what you do wear day to day to ensure functionality in movement. Loose-fitting clothing and sensible shoes can be adapted to almost any situation. Before you put something on, ask yourself, "If I really needed to, would I be able to sprint and climb a wall in this?"

SAFETY

Parkour is not a dangerous activity if you progress slowly, do not take unnecessary risks, and learn the correct safety techniques.

SAFETY TAP

The safety tap is a technique that helps prevent injuries when landing on your feet.

It is good for those times when rolling may not be possible because of a lack of room or other factors, although it's best to use rolls when dropping from greater heights and/or on angles.

To do the safety tap, drop down from a ledge. Start with small drops and work your way up as your confidence builds.

Land on the balls of both feet at the same time, and then roll your heels down towards the ground.

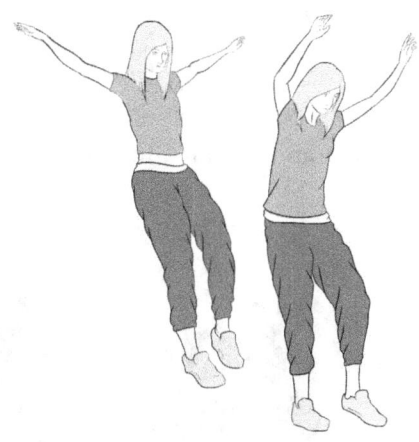

Bend your knees as you land to absorb the shock. Depending on the impact, you can go all the way into a crouch.

Don't slam your wrists down. They are used for assistance and/or balance, but should not be sustaining any major impact.

Spring back up, using the momentum to continue your run.

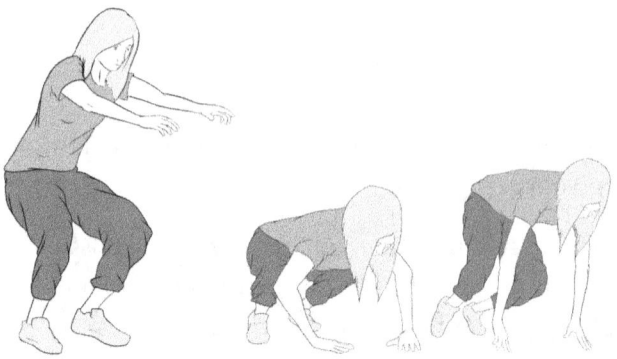

Try to land as softly and quietly as possible. This is true with most things in parkour. The quieter you are, the softer you are, and the less pressure you put on your joints. Since the practical use for parkour is to run from your enemy, it is also advantageous to be as silent as possible.

When dropping down from a wall (e.g., from a cat hang, for example), it's a good idea to turn away from the obstacle. You may have to use your feet to push away from the wall a little so you can get the room to turn.

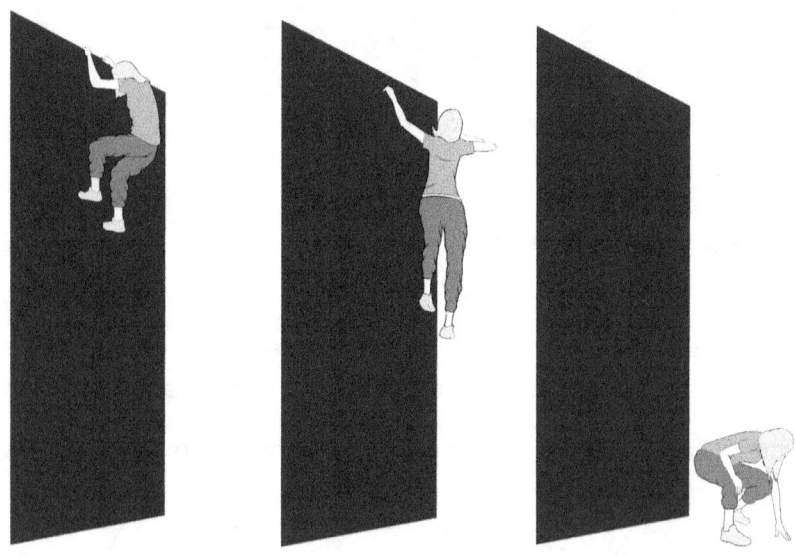

SAFETY ROLLS

The safety roll is an extremely important parkour skill to develop. It is used to prevent injury from a technique gone wrong, a big drop, a general fall or trip, and/or from someone throwing/pushing you to the ground or off something. It's also a good technique for transitioning between movements.

Your aim should be to make your safety roll instinctive. This is because the times you will need it most are those when you are not ready.

The safety roll can be done forwards, sideways, or backwards. You'll probably use the forward roll most often, but you should practice all of them regularly.

When you're first learning the safety roll, do it on soft ground, such as on grass, mats, or sand. Take it slow and start low. Once you have the technique, you can progress by increasing height and/or momentum.

Forward Roll

Choose which side you are most comfortable rolling over, right or left. Eventually, you'll want to learn to roll on both sides.

If rolling over your left shoulder, start from a kneeling position with your left foot forward.

Place your hands on the ground in front of you, so that your thumbs and index fingers form a kind of diamond shape. Put them at a 45° angle in the direction that you want to roll in.

Note: You could just roll over your shoulder, but unless you have something in your hands it's preferable to use them to help control your motion, as well as to absorb some of the impact.

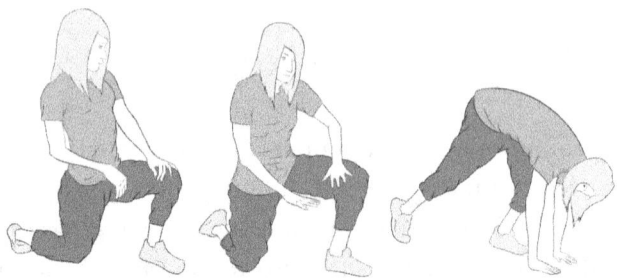

Look over your right shoulder and use your rear leg to push you over into the roll. Use your hands to control your momentum and your arms to lift you a little, so that you can land on the back of your shoulder blade. You do not want to hit on the top of your shoulder.

Roll diagonally across your back to your opposite hip. If you roll wrong (which you probably will when first learning), you'll feel it. When you start practicing on hard surfaces, you will definitely know if you're rolling poorly. It's a learning curve.

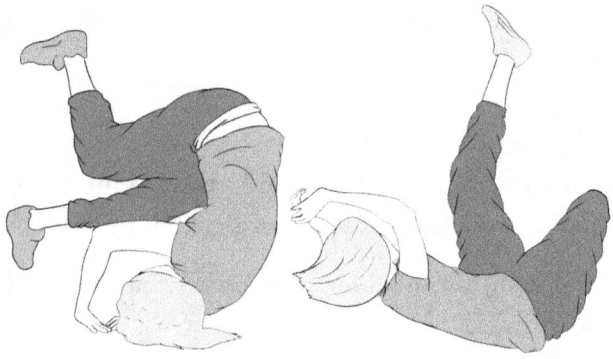

Come up from your roll between your tail and hip bones, and use the side of your leg and your momentum to get back onto your feet.

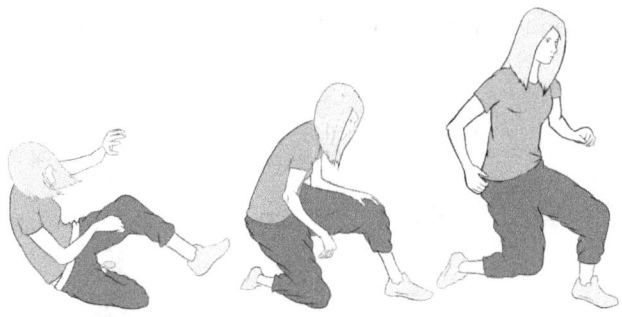

You could also come straight up onto your feet instead of using your thigh. This will save your knee from contacting the ground, but puts more pressure on your ankle as you stand.

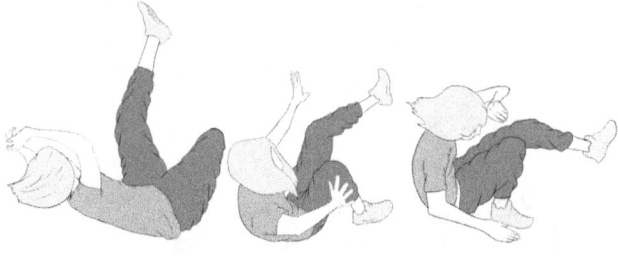

As you get more confident, start from taller positions such as squatting and standing. A good exercise is to stand straight and let your body fall forward like a plank.

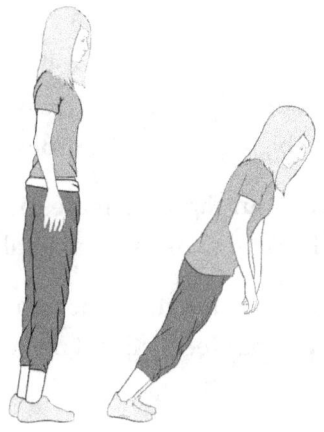

At the last moment, roll out of it. This can be done with side and back rolls as well.

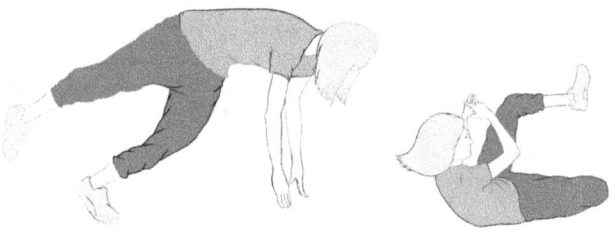

Progress to rolling with momentum and with jumps. When jumping into a roll, be sure to keep your legs flexed as you land and allow the momentum to push you into the roll.

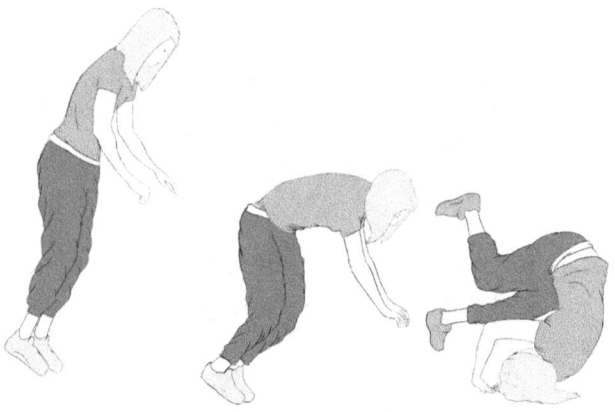

Eventually you will be able to jump and roll from ledges. It is important to slowly work your way up and increase the strength in your legs so that you can do bigger and bigger drops.

As height and speed of your drops increases, it will help to land with your feet closer together and to be more adaptable with your arms.

Note: Dropping into a roll is not the same as a dive roll. When you're dropping from a height, your feet will still make contact first.

Side Roll

The side roll is good for preventing injury when falling in a weird direction.

The technique is very similar to that of a forward roll, except that you will roll on a more horizontal angle across your back. The exact rolling path will also depend on the angle you are falling at.

As you fall, use your hands to help control your movement. Ensure that you clear your arm/shoulder and land somewhere on your back.

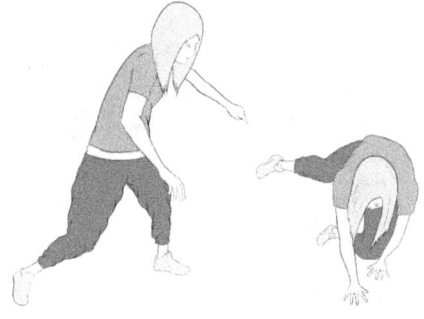

Use the momentum to create as smooth a roll as possible, and then come back onto your feet.

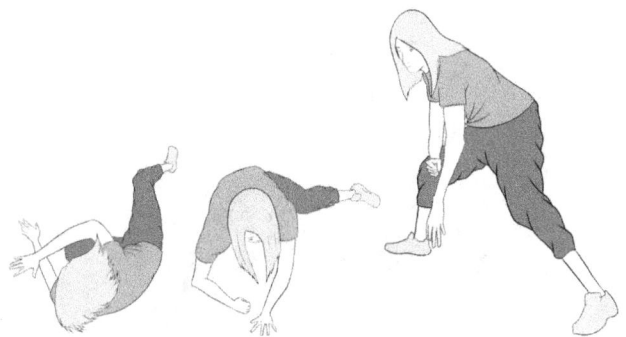

Back Roll

When you're first learning the back roll, it helps to do the forward roll first. Do the forward roll and stop before getting to your feet, then roll back using the same line as you rolled forward on.

Roll forward and back a few times to get the feeling.

When you're ready, you can back roll and come up to stand. At the end of your back roll, continue to go over your shoulder.

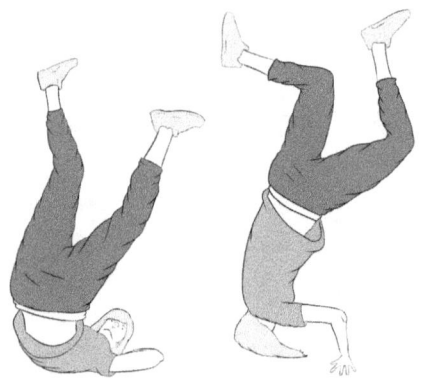

Use your hands to push yourself up a little so you can get onto your feet.

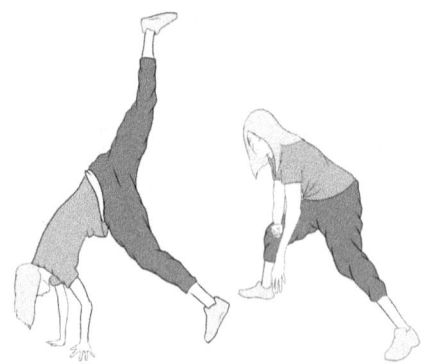

When you're back rolling from a drop, always try to get absorb the landing with your legs as much as possible. Landing with one foot in behind the other will make going into the roll much easier.

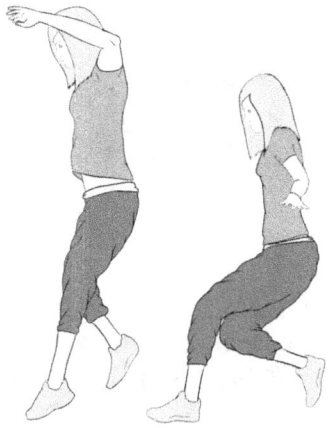

Lower yourself down as much as possible and then go into the roll.

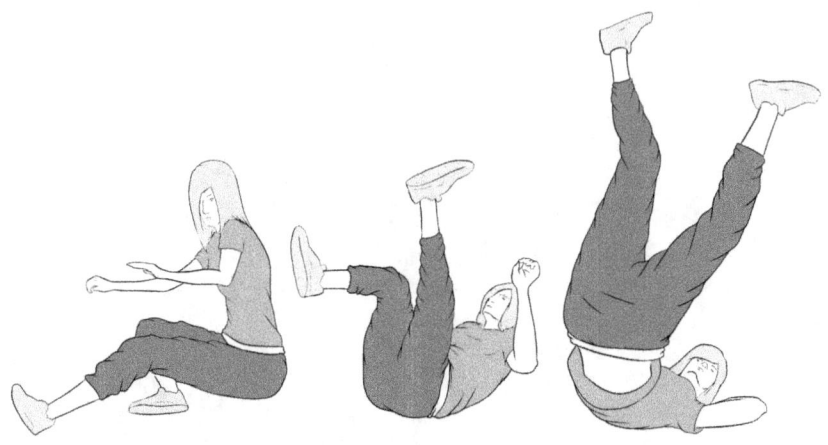

Get back to your feet as previously described.

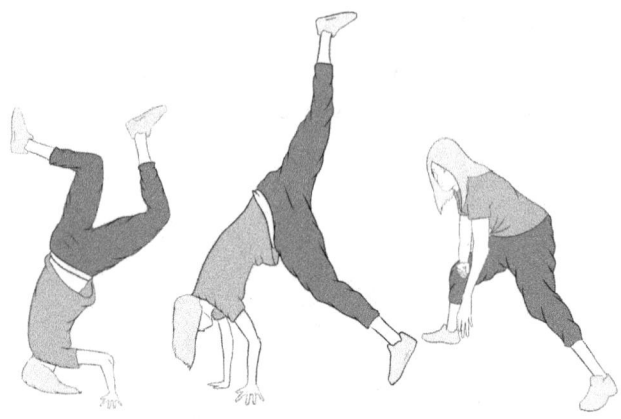

It is important to practice rolling until it's an instinctive reaction, and then to continue to practice it regularly with all variations (jumping, momentum, both sides of the body, landing at different angles, etc.).

Related Chapters:

- Dive Roll

BREAK-FALLING

Break-falling is primarily a martial arts technique used to lessen the impact when you fall. It's not very conducive to parkour because it disrupts "flow"—once you break-fall, you stop—but it's necessary to learn for safety reasons.

Break-falling works by spreading the impact of the fall across a larger portion of your body. It may still hurt a little, but much less damage will be done.

Rolling is always preferable to break-falling, since it's also a quick way to get back on your feet. However, there will be times when the safety roll is not feasible, such as when there's a lack of space. This is when the break-fall comes in very handy.

There are a few different ways to break-fall. In the Survival Fitness Plan, the judo method is used, because judo is a martial art that makes heavy use of throwing people to the ground. Therefore, they really need to know how to break-fall well.

Note: After any break-fall, you can return to your feet with the safety roll, or just use your hands to help you stand.

Practice break-falling on soft ground, such as grass, gym mats, sand, etc. It will also help to breathe out as you hit the ground.

In all break-falls, there are two big things to watch out for.

1. Do not stick your hand down. For many people, this is a natural reaction when falling, but doing it will focus the impact of the fall onto a single point, which is likely to cause injury.
2. Protect your head from hitting the ground. This is done differently depending on the break-fall, but the basic idea is to move your head or face away from the ground.

Back Break-Fall

Stand with your feet about shoulder-width apart.

Squat down as low as you can and tuck your chin to your chest. Tucking your chin will keep you from hitting the back of your head on the ground.

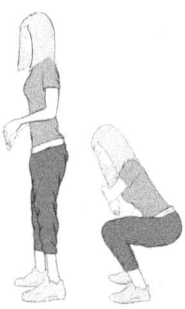

Fall onto your back and arms, allowing a slight roll, but don't roll back too much.

If you stop the roll "dead," it will put too much pressure on your body, but you don't want your legs to go too far towards your head for the same reason.

Having your feet turned out a little and your knees slightly bent will help you to control this.

Your arms will splay out at about 45°.

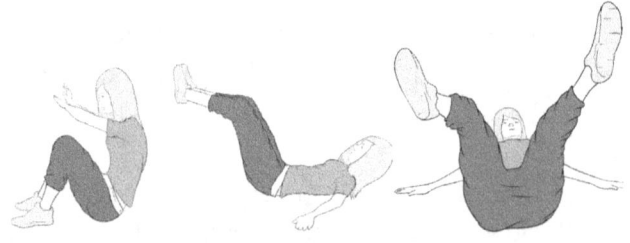

Side Break-Fall

From a standing position, step forward with your right leg and do a single-leg squat as you bring your left leg through. The more you bend the leg, the closer you'll be to the ground before landing.

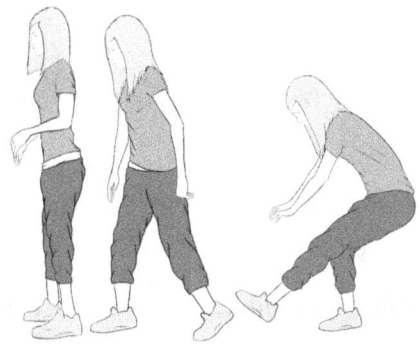

Get as low to the ground as you can, tuck your chin to your chest, and then fall onto the left side of your torso/back and on the whole of your left arm at about a 45° angle from your body, palm facing down. Your legs will probably go in the air.

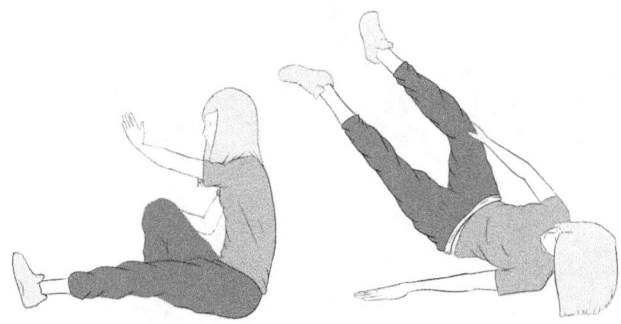

Allow your legs to come back to the ground, finishing in a comfortable position, but not splayed too wide or crossed.

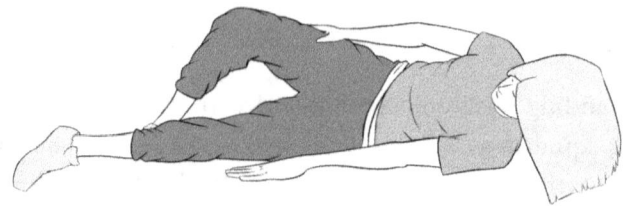

Forward Break-Fall

With the front break-fall, you fall directly forward and land on your forearms.

Start on your knees so you're low to the ground. Put your arms in front of your face in an upside-down V.

As you fall towards the ground, tense your core and take the impact on your forearms. Try not to let your belly hit the ground and turn your face to the side.

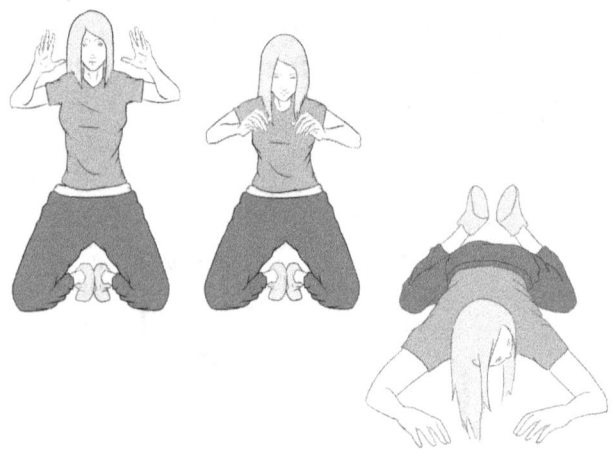

Once you are confident, do this from a standing position. Spread your legs so you can be lower to the ground.

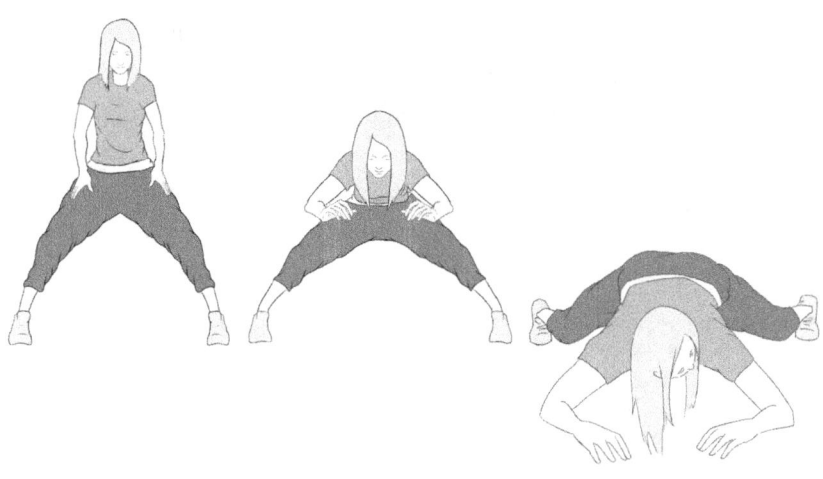

Eventually, you'll be able to do it from a full standing position and with a little jump.

Forward Roll Break-Fall

The forward roll break-fall is useful to know when you go to roll but there is an obstacle ahead preventing you from standing up.

Do a forward safety roll as normal, but instead of coming onto your feet, stop in the side break-fall position.

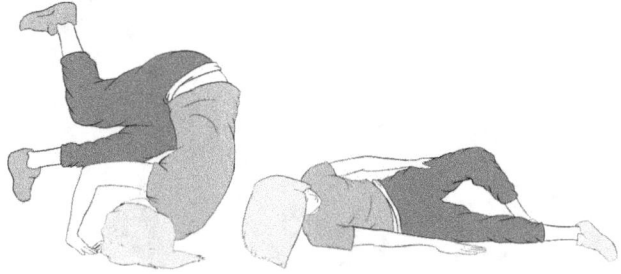

From there, you can do a backwards safety roll to get back to your feet.

With all break-falls, once you're confident in your technique, you can try doing them with less and less of a squat. You can also try them in different scenarios, such as falling off a chair.

Related Chapters:

- Safety Rolls

WARM-UPS AND CONDITIONING

Use warm-up exercises to prepare your body for vigorous activity. A proper warm-up is essential to prevent injury.

Conditioning will strengthen your muscles and improve endurance.

Most of the exercises in this section are both warm-up and conditioning rolled into one.

They are all also useful as parkour movements in their own right, as well as being "stepping stones" to the more advanced parkour techniques outlined in this manual.

CATWALK

The catwalk is a form of quadrupedal movement. Quadrupedal movement is the act of moving on all fours. Other types of quadrupedal movement described in this book include side sapiens and ground kongs.

All types of quadrupedal movement have their practical uses, and they also make great warm-up/conditioning exercises.

The catwalk is useful when you have to traverse ledges, rails, etc., or to get through or under small areas. It gives you more balance and control on the obstacle, and it lowers your profile, which makes it great to use for escape and evasion.

Start by getting down on your hands (flat palms) and feet, with your left hand in front of your right hand, and your right foot in front of your left foot. Your hands and feet should form a line. As you move forward you want to maintain this line as much as possible. When you're first starting, it will help to follow an actual line on the ground. When you're on a ledge or rail, you will have little choice anyway.

To move forward, first move your rear hand to the front, then your rear foot to the front. Repeat this. Start slowly, with small steps, and ensure that you transfer the weight evenly between your arm and legs —front and back, left and right.

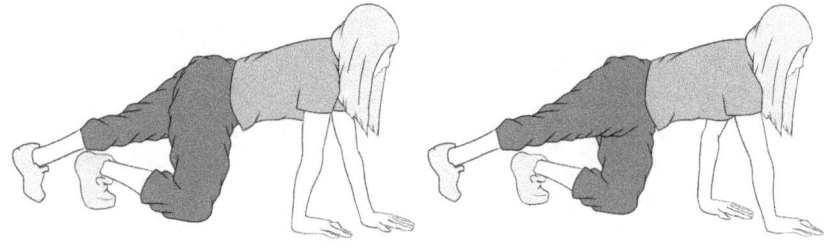

For stability, keep three points of contact with the surface at all times.

Once your movement is coordinated, concentrate on perfecting your posture. Make yourself as level as possible, from your hips to your head. Keep your back flat and your head forward.

Don't stretch yourself out, bring your knees too close to your body, or stick your bum out.

When you need a rest, crouch. Do not put your knees on the ground.

Progress further and work different muscles by cat-walking backwards, up and down stairs, getting really low, on ledges, on rails, etc.

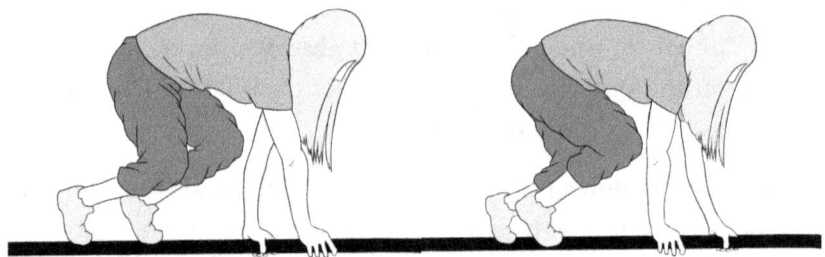

Related Chapters:

- Side Sapiens
- Ground Kongs

BALANCE

Balance is very important in parkour. One way to improve it is with rail work, or doing various exercises on a rail. There are a couple described in this chapter, but you can create your own also. Rail work also has other advantages, such as:

- Building resilient joints to help sustain the stresses of high-impact jumping and landing.
- Cultivating body awareness.
- Improving all-over body strength.
- Increasing your focus levels.

Ideally, you'll want to be able to do all these exercises on a round rail since it is (in most places) the hardest, most common urban structure to balance on. Progress to this by starting on the ground, then moving to ledges, flat planks, square rails, etc.

Squatting

First, you need to be able to get into the squat position on the ground.

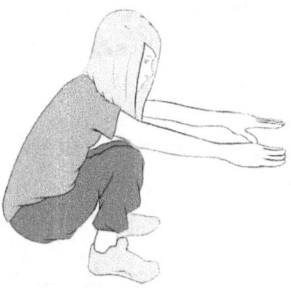

If you do not have the flexibility for this, use the seated forward bend and downward dog to improve it. You can find instructions to these stretches in the General Health and Fitness section of this book.

Rail Squat

Once you can do at least ten squats on the ground, try them on the rail. You can hold onto it to start with. When you've found your balance/confidence, let go. It may help to focus your gaze on a single point in front of you.

Stand slowly. Keep standing on the rail for a few seconds. Once you're ready, go down and up again.

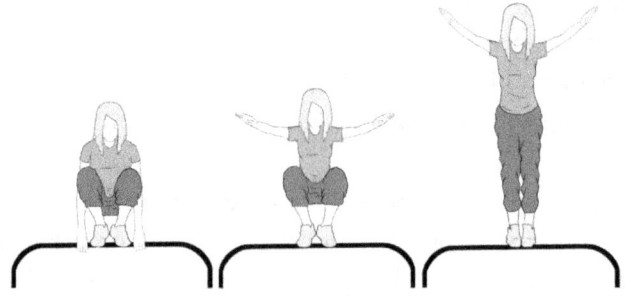

Rail Walk

The next step is to walk. Walk forward a bit, then turn around and walk back.

It will help to start on something easier than a rail. At the most basic level, you can just follow a line on the ground, then use a wide plank and thinner ones as you progress.

The key to keeping balance is correct posture. As you walk, keep your chest up, knees slightly bent, and your bum over your heels. Take each step toes first.

Go slowly to begin with, use "airplane arms" until you're confident, and stop to regain balance when needed.

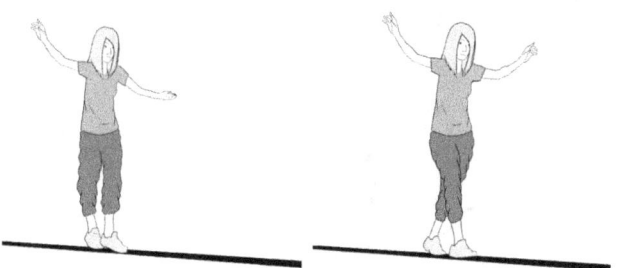

Try walking backwards as well.

Note: In a real-life scenario, you would most likely use a monkey traverse or catwalk on the rail, as these two methods would give you more control and a lower profile.

Rail Balance Routine

Once you can do all the things above, you can put them into a short rail-balancing routine that you can do regularly. Jump up on to the rail, get balanced in the squat position, do a few squats on the rail, stand, walk forward, turn around, walk backwards, and catwalk. Increase difficulty with inclined rails.

Slacklining

When you want to become a beast of balance, you can move from the rail to slacklining. Just do the rail balancing routine on the slackline.

Slacklining is basically tightrope walking but most people will use a dynamic (stretchy), flat, broad (a few inches) piece of webbing tied between two anchor points, usually trees.

To learn more about slackening, including the various types and how to set a line up, visit:

Slackline.hivefly.com/slacklining-for-beginners-step-by-step

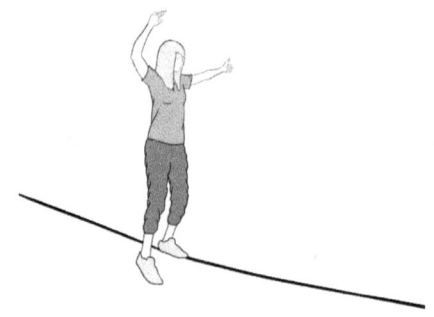

Related Chapters:

- Downward Dog
- Seated Forward Bend
- Catwalk
- Monkey Traverse

SIDE SAPIENS

Side sapiens (a.k.a. side monkeys) are a type of quadrupedal movement that are used as a progression to the reverse vault.

They are also useful in their own right as a way to displace momentum (such as when you're landing from a drop) and/or to continue flow into your next movement.

Start in a low squat position.

Reach your arms out across your body to your left and plant them firmly on the ground. Your right hand should land first, followed closely by your left.

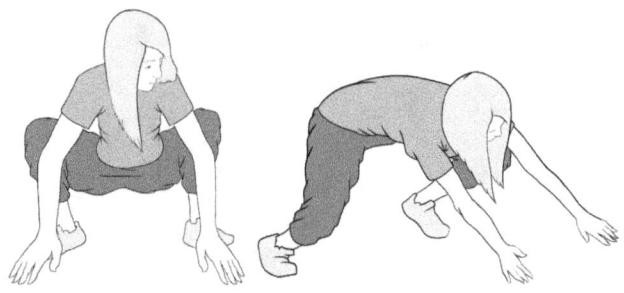

Keep your arms strong and use them to support your body weight as you bring your legs to your left. Your right foot should land first, followed closely by your left, so that you end up back in the low squat position.

Engage your core and land with control. Land lightly with your feet and as quietly as you can.

Repeat this movement a few times and then go back the other way.

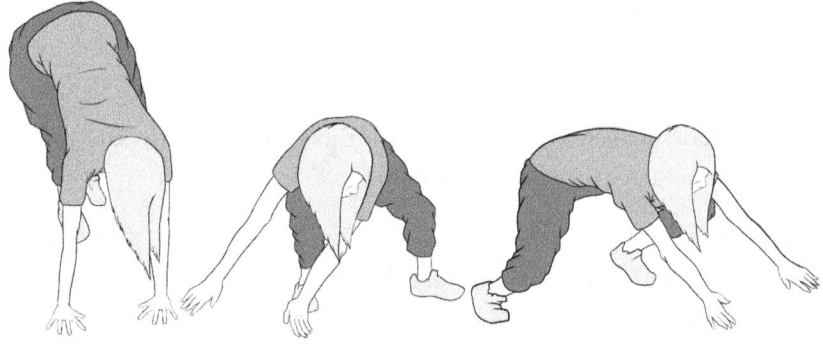

This is also good to practice on ledges and rails.

For more of a challenge, you can do this exercise with straight legs.

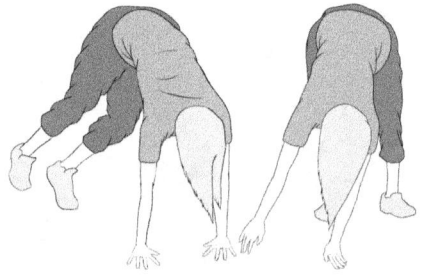

Related Chapters:

- Reverse Vault

GROUND KONGS

Ground kongs are a type of quadrupedal movement used as a progression to the kong vault.

They are also useful in their own right as a way for you to displace momentum (such as when you're landing from a drop) and/or to continue flow into your next movement.

Start in a low squat position.

Reach forward and plant both your hands firmly on the ground.

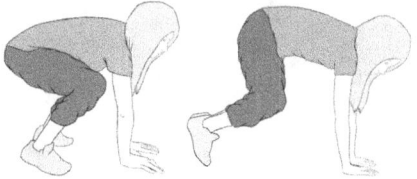

Keep your arms strong and use them to support your body weight as you bring your legs up to your hands (or as close as you can).

Engage your core and land with control. Land lightly with your feet and as quietly as you can.

Repeat this movement a few times.

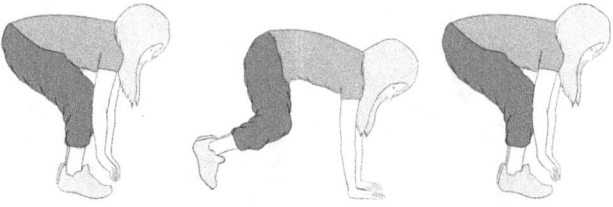

When you are confident, practice on ledges and rails. As you build strength you can try to cover more ground.

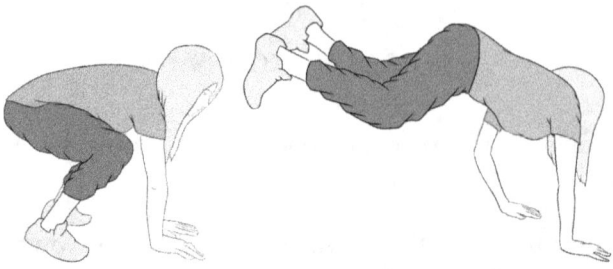

You can also do ground kongs backwards which will target a different set of muscles.

Related Chapters:

- Kong Vault

PULL-UPS

Pull-ups are an excellent all-body exercise. Doing them regularly will help condition you for wall climb-ups and, eventually, muscle-ups.

Grab the bar with a grip slightly wider than shoulder-width apart and with your palms facing away from you.

Let yourself hang all the way down.

Pull yourself up by pulling your shoulder blades down and together. Keep your chest up and pull up until your chin is above the bar. Touch your chest to it.

As you are pulling up, keep your body in a vertical line. Do not swing. Concentrate on isolating your back and biceps.

Pause at the top, and then lower yourself back down into the hanging position.

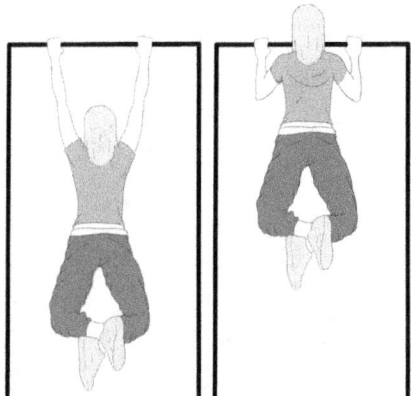

Related Chapters:

- Wall Climb-up
- Muscle-ups

RUNNING AND JUMPING

This section contains techniques to do with running and jumping over or between obstacles without coming into contact with them. It also includes explanations of parkour runs and games.

SPRINTING

In parkour, you sprint in between overcoming obstacles.

Sprinting is an efficient form of exercise. It's far more effective to do multiple short sprints than it is to run/jog long distance. Sprinting gives the same health benefits in a much shorter time, as well as other benefits that jogging or running do not offer.

Unlike jogging or running, sprinting creates explosive power, which is very important in parkour. Sprinting is very functional and much more useful than long-distance jogging when it comes to escaping from danger.

If for some reason you do need to run for a long distance, practicing parkour in general you will give you the endurance you need to do so —more than you would have if you just went jogging every day.

Proper Running Technique

Using proper running technique will enable you to go faster and longer while expending less energy.

When running (sprinting), keep your elbows bent at 90° and move your hand from your pocket to your chin.

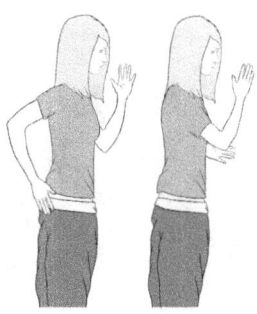

Move your knees and elbows in unison. As you drive your elbows back, bring your knees up. Then, as your hand goes to your chin, drive your leg back down.

Be sure to bring your hand from your pocket to your chin. The further back your elbows go, the higher your knees will go.

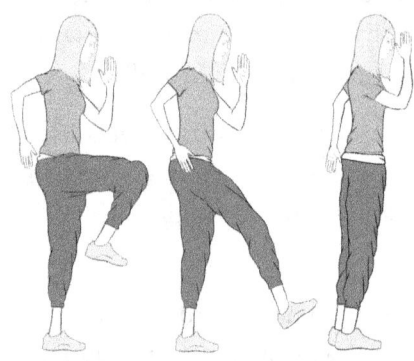

Keep your chin level, eyes focused forward, core engaged, shoulders relaxed, and torso upright (opposed to leaning forward).

This posture keeps your mass vertical, which means your feet will strike the ground with more force and you will produce more speed.

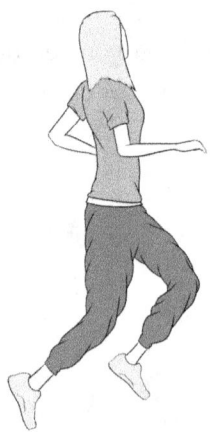

Even when you get tired, always keep correct running form.

Mouth Breathing

You use up a lot of oxygen while running, which you need to replace efficiently.

Breathing through your mouth allows more oxygen to enter your body. It also prevents you from clenching your teeth together, which may cause headaches.

Note: When you're breathing normally, or if you have to run in high pollution, it is better to breathe through your nose. Your nose is your body's air treatment system. It filters, humidifies, and warms the air before it reaches the rest of your body.

Belly Breathing

Learn this first by lying on your back. As you exhale, use your stomach muscles to help expel all the air from your lungs. To inhale, just relax your stomach muscles and let the air come in.

Once you're comfortable with belly breathing, use it while sprinting.

Breathing in Step

Breathing in time to your steps is the easiest way to regulate the rhythm of your breath. This is useful for monitoring and controlling certain things while you are running.

At a normal run rate (not sprinting), stay at a 2:2 ratio. That is, inhale over two steps and then exhale over two steps. During harder runs, you may need to change the ratio to 1:2 or 2:1.

When you go up a hill, maintain the same breath ratio as you were using before the hill. This ensures you'll use the same amount of energy to get over the hill.

To fix a side-stitch while running, slow your breathing to a deeper 3:3 rhythm.

Another way to fix a stitch is to expand and contract your diaphragm in the opposite direction from usual. When you breathe in, make your stomach contract, and when you exhale make your stomach expand.

Note: Breathing at a 1:1 ratio or faster may lead to hyperventilation, and breathing at a 3:3 ratio or slower means you may not get enough oxygen into your body.

EVASIVE RUNNING

Evasive running is the ability to maneuver out of the way of an oncoming or stationary obstacle while running.

When learning evasive running, use a running speed slightly slower than sprinting. You want to be quick, but not so quick that you will get injured while performing the movement.

Train to evade humans, as they will be the hardest to outsmarting. You want to go in whichever direction is hardest for your opponent to go.

As you approach your opponent, look him in the eye. This will make it harder for him to predict where you are going, and he will probably think you're charging straight at him.

If your opponent is square on with you but is flat-footed (left picture), it should be fairly easy to pass him on either side.

If he has one side forward more (right image), evade him by going to the other side of his body. It will probably be his weaker side, and it will be harder for him to maneuver in that direction. In the scenario in the picture on the right, you would maneuver to the woman's left. since her right foot is forward.

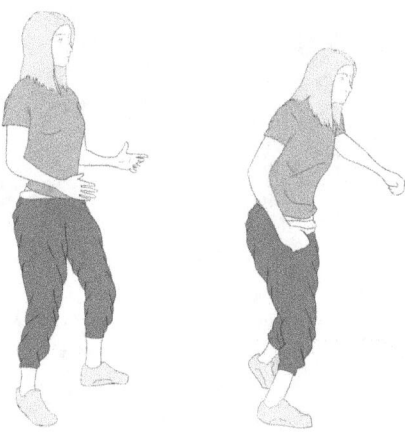

If an opponent angles away from you, then go the opposite way. In the picture, the woman has stepped to her left with her right foot.

You would evade her by moving to her right, to the outside of her.

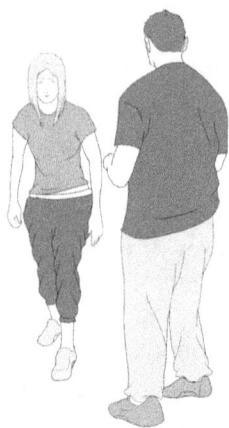

You can practice this with a friend. Have your friend face you square on as you run towards him.

When you are close, your friend should step toward you and you should evade in the best direction.

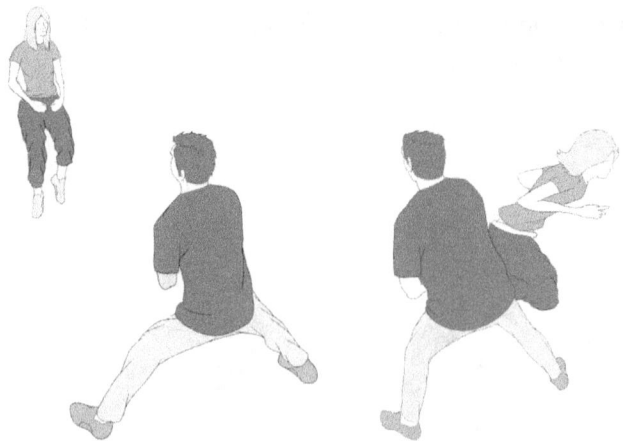

You could also practice against a stationary object. Run towards it and evade it on either side at the last moment.

Related Chapters:

- Sprinting

HURDLES

Hurdles are often neglected in parkour, but they are the fastest way to pass an obstacle, and sometimes—if you're dealing with chain-link fences or hedges, for example—the only way. You should use them whenever possible. They are best used over small obstacles that you are confident you can clear.

The mechanics of hurdles can be learned with a couple of drills.

Trail Leg Drill

The trail leg drill teaches you to lift your rear leg up and to the outside as opposed to coming straight through.

Face a wall just over one natural step away, and lean your palms flat against it. Bring your left leg straight up behind you and then bring your knee to the front, parallel to your hip.

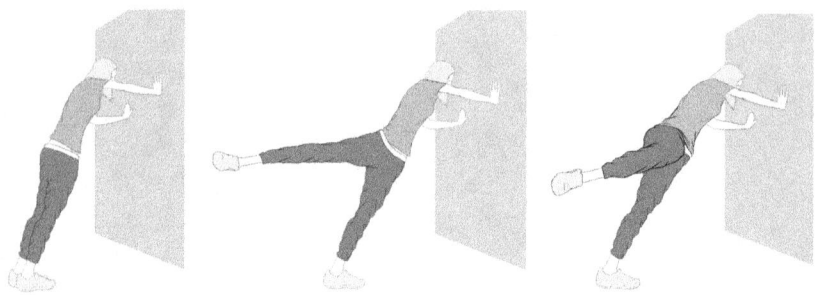

Keep your heel directly behind your knee far as you can, and then snap your foot back down to the ground.

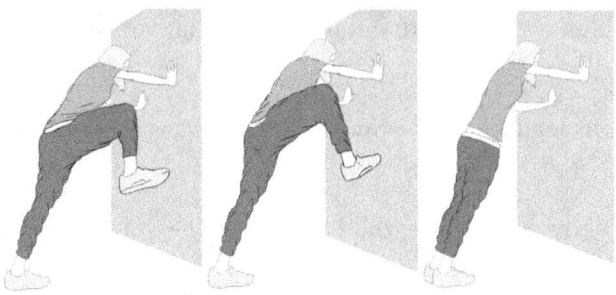

Do this drill ten times on each side of your body.

Front-Leg Drill

The front-leg drill teaches you to lean forward which is very important for momentum.

Stand facing a wall, just over one natural step away from it.

Thrust your front leg straight up and into the wall. Really lean into it. As you bring your leg up, reach forward with your opposite hand.

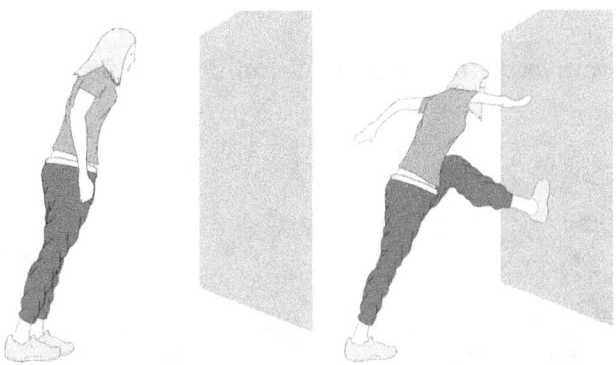

Do this drill ten times on each side of your body.

The Hurdle

After you have practiced those two drills, you can try an actual hurdle.

Approach an obstacle with enough speed that you're confident you'll clear it.

Thrust your lead foot and opposite arm forward as you kick your rear leg back.

As your body comes over the obstacle, bring your rear knee to the front, parallel to your hip.

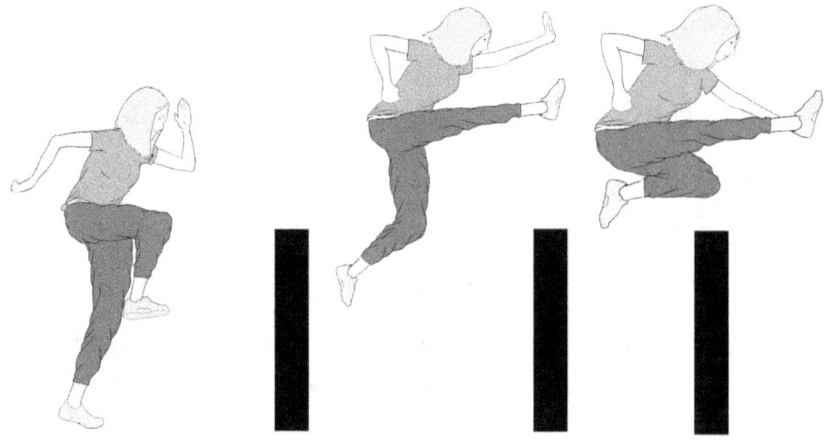

Land on your lead foot and continue running forward.

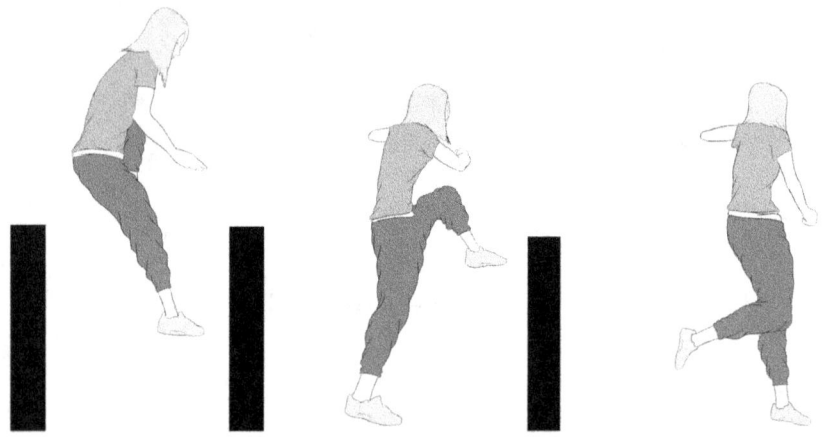

PRECISION JUMPING

Precision jumping is a fundamental parkour skill in which you jump from one stationary point to another. It is important to learn how to be precise with your landings so that you can land safely on smaller obstacles such as ledges, handrails, and walls.

When you're doing precision jumping, your aim is to land exactly on your intended landing spot, with no extra momentum in either direction—that is, without stumbling forward.

Begin with your feet together and bend your knees a little, so you're in a semi-crouched position.

Move your arms behind you as you shift your weight to the balls of your feet.

Lean forward. The greater the distance you need to jump, the more you need to lean.

As you jump, throw your arms forwards and upwards. Your energy will travel up your legs, through your torso, and into your hands.

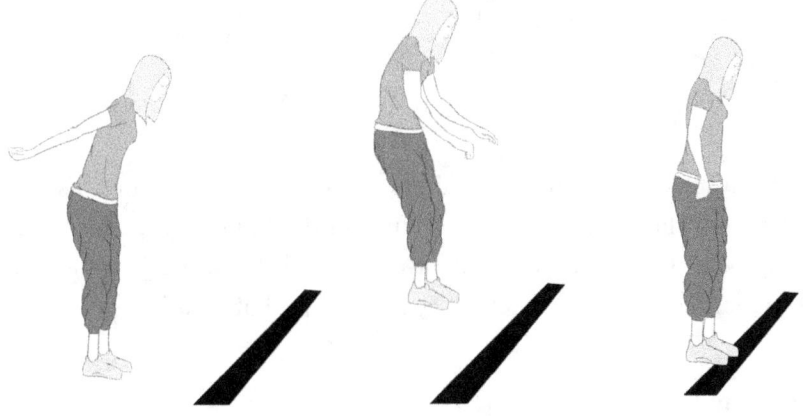

Aim to arc up and then come down on to the landing area, landing on the balls of your feet as quietly as you can. Land on both feet at the same time, just as you would in the safety tap.

As you build confidence, start jumping from farther back and with small level differences, such as onto a curb.

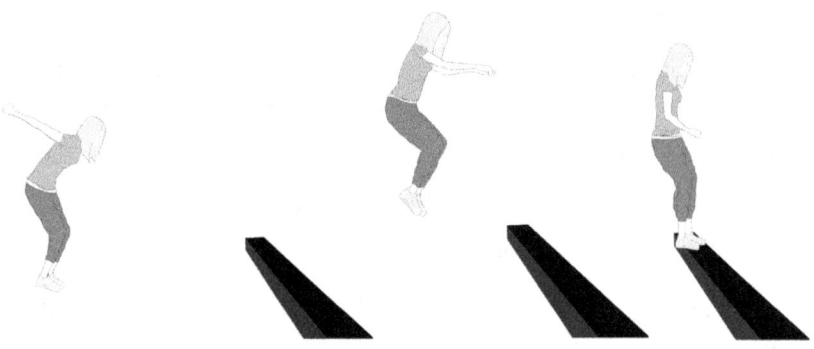

You can also try high to low, to/from rails, etc.

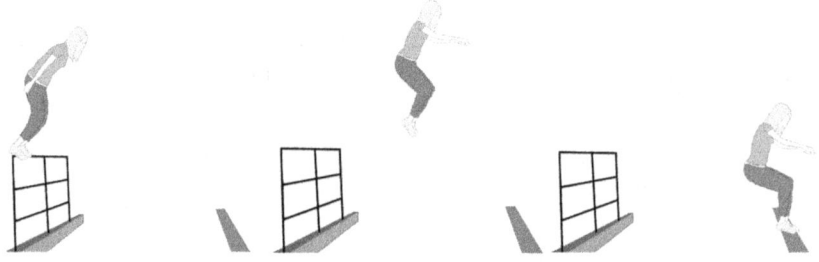

Note: When jumping onto smaller platforms (such as handrails) it is extra important that you aim to land on the balls of your feet. This way, if you slip a little then you have the whole of your foot to recover. If you land on your heels and slip, you will probably fall.

Jumping Larger Gaps

Note: It's a good idea to learn the crane landing before attempting larger gaps just in case you jump short.

Practice precision jumping over larger gaps on the ground first to see if you can make it. This is also useful to improve your distance.

Use lines on the road or any other type of marker, so you can take off and land on exact points.

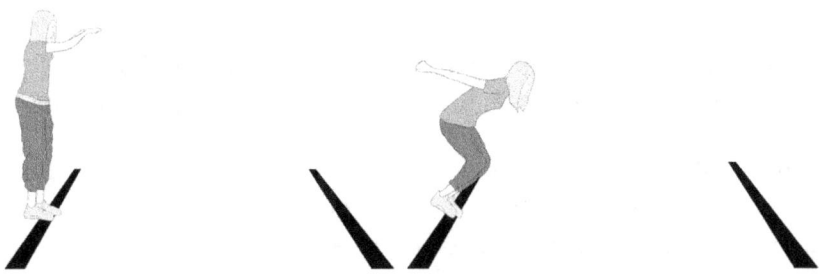

When doing longer precision jumps, focus more on extending your body. Once you are in the air, bring your knees forward.

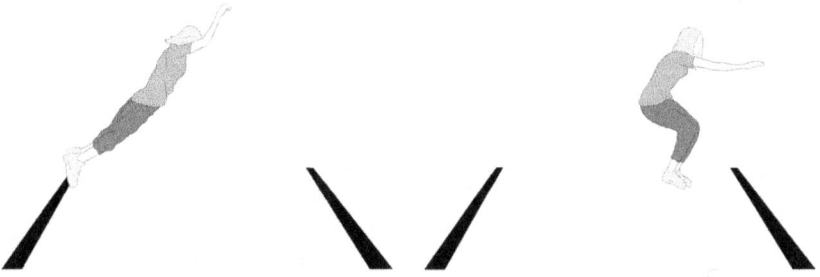

Push your feet towards the landing point and land as softly as you can.

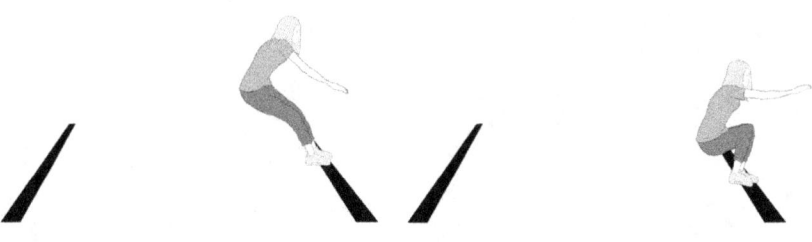

Running Precision Jumps

When precision jumping over very large gaps, you can use the running precision jump. The running precision jump is exactly what it sounds like—a precision jump with a run up, as opposed to leaping from a stationary position.

The running precision jump uses a one-foot take off, but you still land with both feet, in the same way as in a standing precision jump.

Since you are jumping with much more momentum, sticking the landing becomes more difficult. Many people find they jump too far and/or stumble forward when landing.

Related Chapters:

- Safety Tap
- Crane Landing

CRANE LANDING

The crane landing is used when you want to land on obstacles that are just a bit too far (either in height or distance) to precision jump onto, but are still small enough that you don't feel the need to cat-hang or vault.

Your intention should be to have one of your feet land on top of the obstacle while the other one supports you down the front of it.

Prepare to jump just like you would in a precision jump.

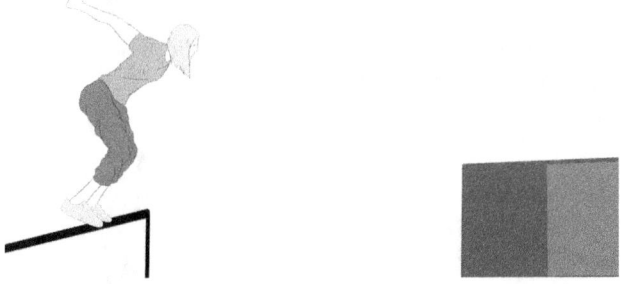

The decision about making a precision jump may be made either before you jump or mid-air.

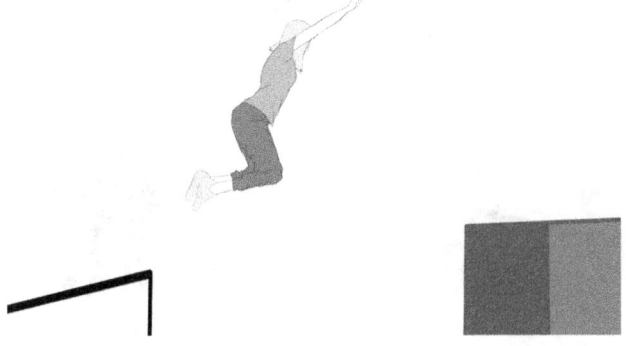

Put the foot that you intend to land on top of the obstacle with in front.

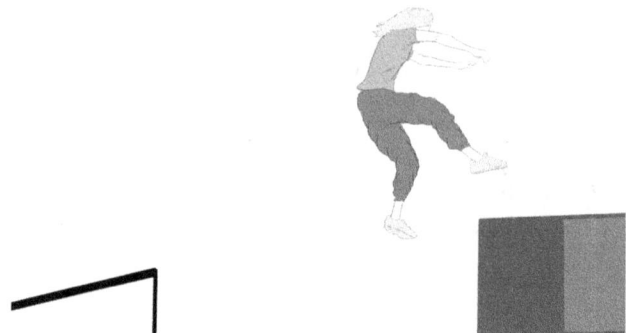

Your front foot should land on top while your rear foot should push against the front of the obstacle to prevent you from falling back.

Once you're stable, bring your rear foot up onto the obstacle.

STRIDING

Parkour striding, a.k.a. bounding, is leaping from one foot to another in succession. It is useful for running across elevated obstacles.

Approach the stride like a running precision jump. Run up and take off from one foot. Stretch your legs out front and back.

As your lead leg lands, you want your center of gravity to be over your foot so you can push off into the next stride.

If you're too far forward or back, it will mess up your momentum.

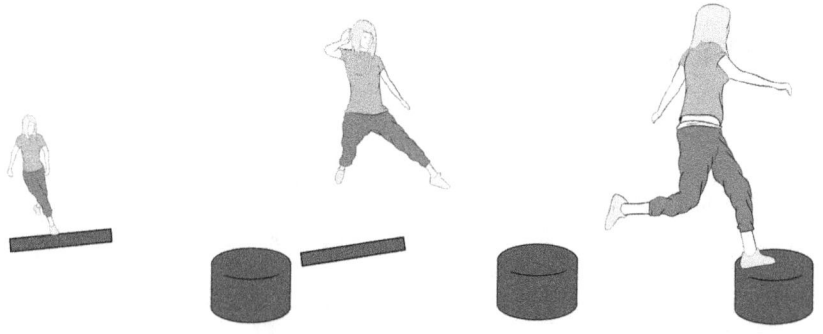

It will help to get your arms and leg in sync, just as you would if you were walking.

You can use this arm swing to generate more power.

The further the distance between your obstacles, the more you should swing your arms.

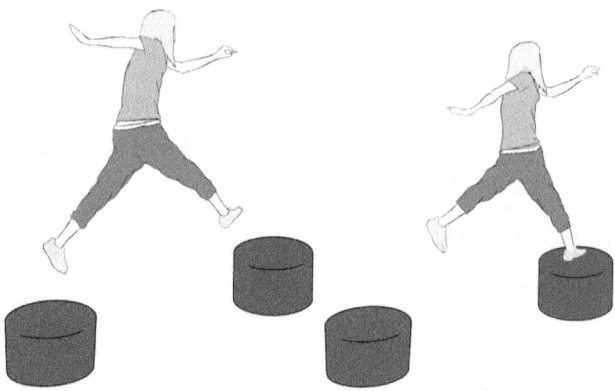

Related Chapters:

- Precision Jumping

STRIDE TO SAFETY STEP

The stride to safety step is used to stride over a gap onto a ledge (or something similar) and then safely move down a level, such as to the ground. It's actually a combination of two other parkour techniques, striding and the safety step-through (a.k.a. down step).

Note: Before you attempt the stride to safety step, you should know how to stride and how to do the safety vault (the safety step-through is covered as part of the safety vault).

Run up to the first ledge and stride off it as usual.

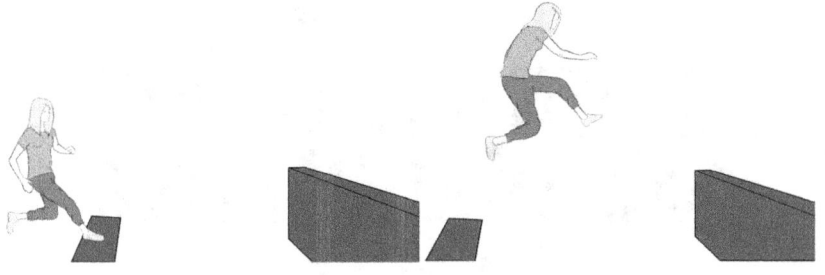

Land on the second ledge one foot first. Most people find it easiest to land on the opposite foot from they took off with, but either foot is possible.

As you land, lean out a little to the opposite side of the foot you landed on. This is so you have enough room for your other leg to come through.

Allow your leg to absorb most of the impact, and then place your hand on the ledge, fingers pointing out to your side.

Your other leg should come through between your hand and foot so you can push yourself away from the edge.

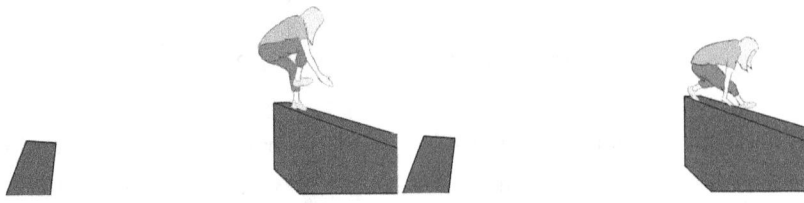

Here is a view from the front.

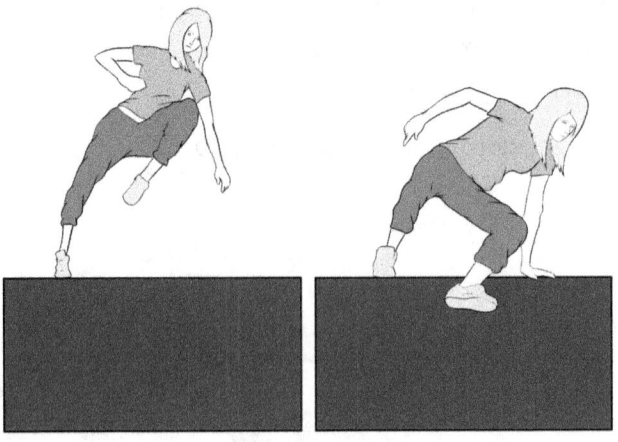

This demonstrates leaving off one leg and then landing on the opposite one, which is the way most people prefer to do it.

You could also leave off one leg and then land on the same one. Experiment to see which you prefer.

It also shows a person going from lower to higher, but you can do it between surfaces of the same level, or from higher to lower.

Related Chapters:

- Striding
- Safety Vault

DIVE ROLL

The dive roll is used to prevent injury when you're coming down on your head.

In most cases, this is intentional in the way of diving over an obstacle, but may also be used in accidental falls where you are low to the ground and don't have the room to land feet-first—if your foot clips on the obstacle while you're hurdling, for example.

Note: In the case that you fell (or were thrown) off something high, landing feet-first and doing a safety roll, if possible, is your best option.

Ensure you are proficient at the safety roll before attempting the dive roll.

Avoid doing the dive roll on hard ground, even when you're proficient.

The technique for doing the dive roll is very similar to the one for the forward roll, but there is a lot more impact and momentum. In addition, you are coming toward your head as opposed to landing on your feet first.

Start by practicing the forward roll from a handstand. You don't need to be great at handstands, you just have to get to the right angle for a moment so you can go into the roll.

Lower yourself with your arms, then lean forward slightly to tuck your head as you go into the roll.

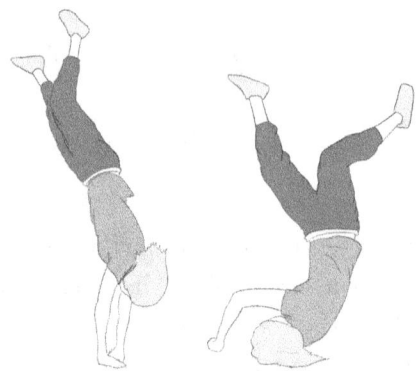

Keep your body strong (arms, core, legs, and neck) as you allow your body to "collapse" into the roll.

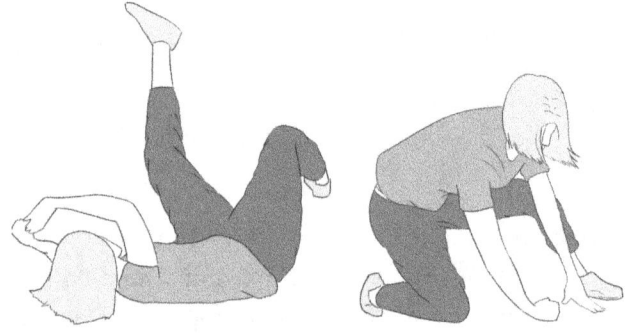

Once you're comfortable, you can start jumping into the dive roll from a standing position.

Kick your leg back as you jump to help get your hips over.

As you hit the ground, absorb some of the impact with your arms by keeping them strong while allowing them to collapse. Use your arms to ensure you get over your head.

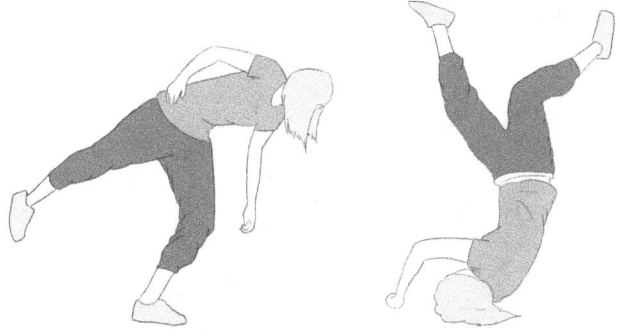

Use the momentum to flow onto your back and into the roll.

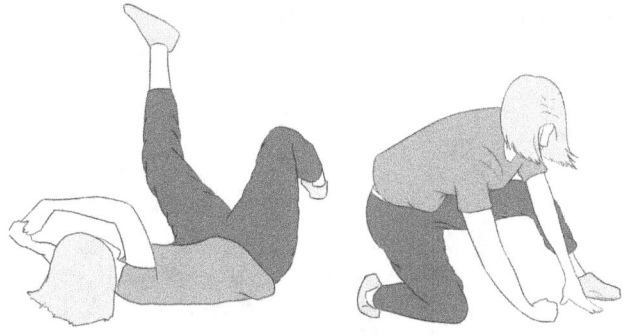

Next try it with a short run up, and then try jumping off with two feet.

Slowly progress until you are doing a full dive roll.

Dive and stretch out like a cat.

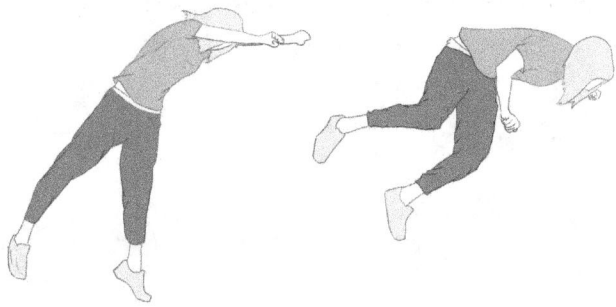

Absorb the impact with your arms.

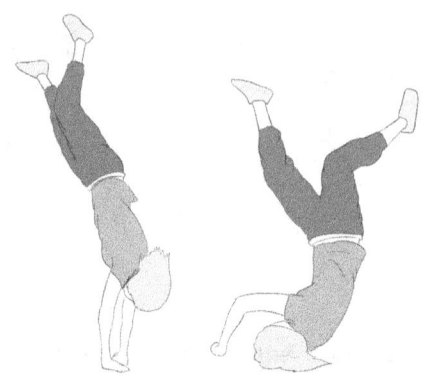

Tuck your head as you go into the roll.

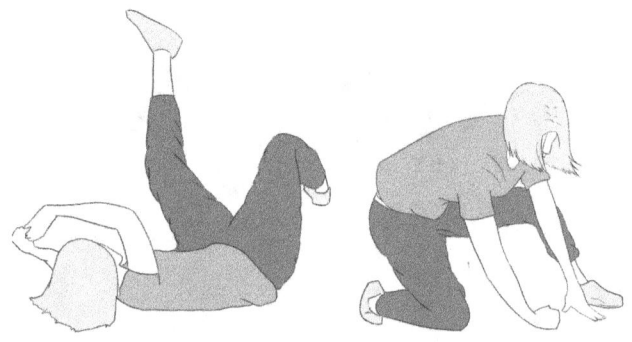

Train at this level until the movement is instinctive, then progress by jumping higher and over things.

When jumping over things, ensure your hips clear the obstacle and your legs/feet follow on the same path.

Related Chapters:

- Safety Rolls

PARKOUR RUNS

A parkour run is when you put your parkour skills into practical use. Basically, the idea is to go from one point to another in the most efficient manner. All you need is a few basic techniques and you can start.

To begin with you may just want to do a short run with two or three techniques put together in a flow. You can suss out a site first so you know exactly what you want to do.

Try different things to see what works best (fastest and most efficiently) for you. Practice each technique individually, and then put them together. Gradually get faster and faster. Eventually you want to be able to go from point A to point B long distance without having to suss it out first.

Good runs are those in which the transition between techniques is smooth. Once you're confident, your aim should be to move as quickly and quietly as possible, adapting to your environment as you go.

PARKOUR GAMES

Parkour games are a good way to vary your training. They are great for kids and adults alike, and most of them are just adaptations of games you probably already know. Here are a couple of examples.

Horse

One person does a technique or short run and the others have to replicate it. If they are unable to replicate it, they get a letter "H." Once they have used up all their letters (HORSE), they are out of the game. Take turns being the person who performs the technique that the others have to replicate.

Of course, the word you spell can be anything, such as PARKOUR.

Quadrupedal Tag

Play a game of tag in which you're only allowed to use different types of quadrupedal movement (ground kongs, side sapiens, cat-walking, etc.). This concept can easily be applied to many other games, such as capture the flag. You can also just play normal tag, but use your parkour skills.

Lava Pit

A childhood favorite where you pretend the ground is molten lava. Move around, being sure not to fall in. This is easily combined with tag.

Related Chapters:

- Side Sapiens

VAULTS

Technically a vault is any type of movement that involves overcoming an obstacle, but in this section it only refers to those movements in which you make contact with the obstacle you are going over.

SAFETY VAULT

The safety vault is used to pass a relatively low and short obstacle in front of you, such as a waist-height wall.

The safety vault is the very first vault learned in Survival Fitness Plan Parkour Training. This is because it is the easiest to learn and the safest to do.

It is also a necessary technique to know so you can progress to the similar but faster speed vault, the reverse safety vault, and the stride-to-safety-step techniques.

An easy way to learn the safety vault is by numbering your hands and feet. It will help you to remember the order of placement.

1. Left hand.
2. Right leg.
3. Left leg.
4. Right hand.

Take it slow to begin with. Get the pattern into your head, and eventually into your muscle memory.

Approach the obstacle and place your left hand (#1) on it. Next, place your right leg (#2). Stretch it out far enough to allow your left leg (#3) to pass between your left hand and right leg.

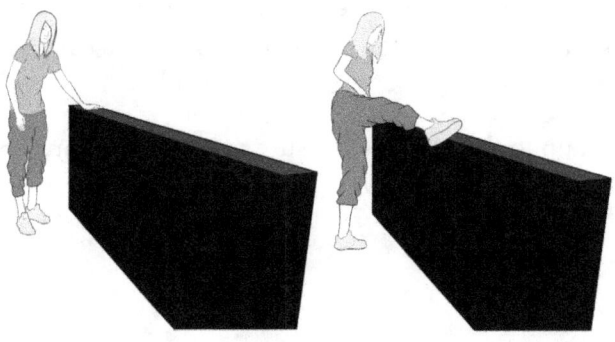

Step straight through with your left leg. Keep your right arm (#4) up so you can pass your leg through easier.

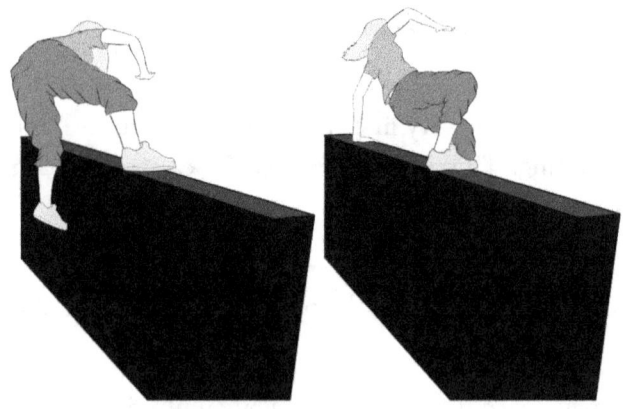

Here is what it looks like from the front.

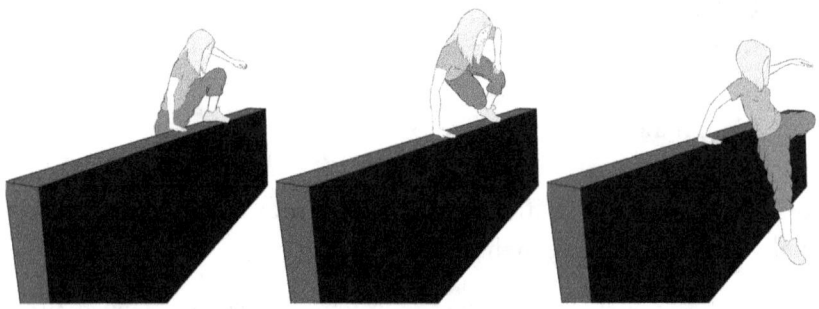

Practice on both sides of your body.

When you add speed, your #1 leg doesn't have to push off that much. It becomes just a touch on top of the obstacle so you can gauge where it is.

As you run up to the obstacle, be sure not to stop in preparation for the vault. Stride directly onto it, and go up and over the object in an arc.

Land with your chest above or in front of your foot, and use your #1 and #2 to push the object behind you so you get more forward momentum. At the same time, reach down to the floor with your #3 leg.

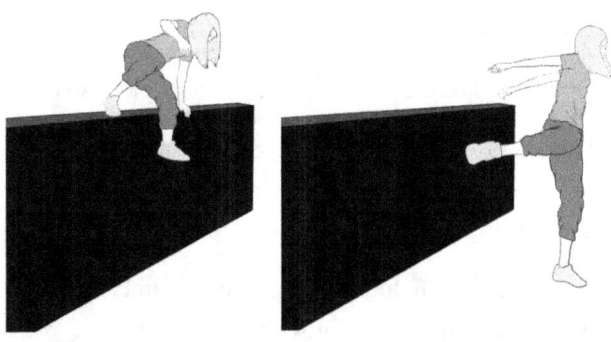

Related Chapters:

- Speed Vault
- Reverse Safety Vault
- Training for Reality

SPEED VAULT

The speed vault is used to quickly pass over small to medium-sized obstacles that are too big for you to hurdle over. Before attempting the speed vault, you should be proficient at the safety vault.

Note: If you're approaching an obstacle at an angle, use the lazy vault.

The speed vault is basically the same as a safety vault, except you don't let your foot touch the wall. You can do the following exercise to get your legs coordinated for this.

If you want to place your left hand on the obstacle, raise your right leg straight out to your right. Quickly follow it with your left. Tap your right foot with your left in the air.

Be sure to raise your right and then your left, as opposed to jumping with both legs at the same time. Your left foot should land back on the ground first.

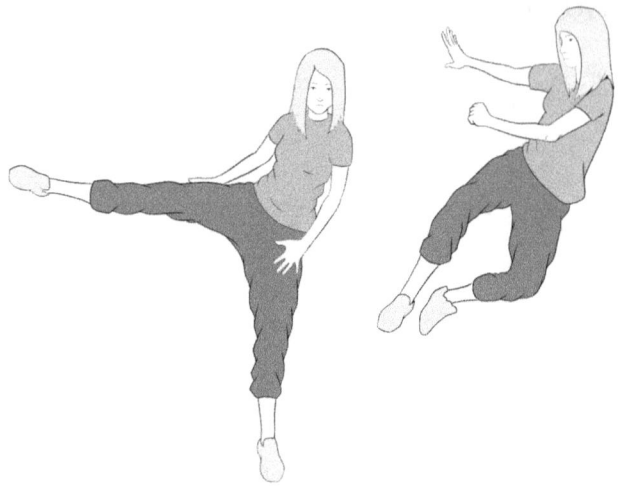

This leg kicking motion is what you use to pass the obstacle, except without tapping your feet.

Approach the object with some speed, so you can clear it. As with most vaults, you want to arc over the obstacle. Run and kick your legs up. Once you're in the air, place your hand on the obstacle (fingers facing forwards) and push up and back to help get your chest and legs through.

Keep your chest pointing forward, and don't hold onto the wall too long; otherwise, it will focus your momentum in a different direction (as opposed to straight ahead).

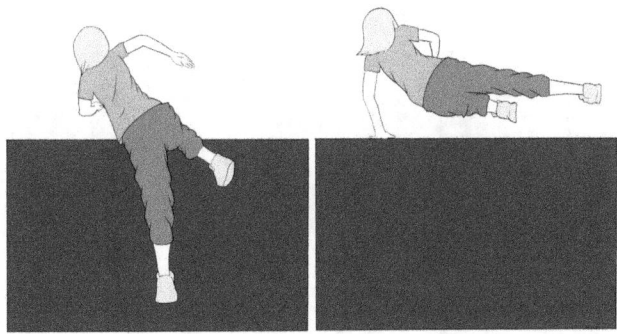

Switch your legs through while you are in the air and land on your inside foot first—that is, the foot on same side as the hand you have on the wall. Your chest should be facing forward and in front of your leading leg as you land. Be sure to push the obstacle behind you before landing.

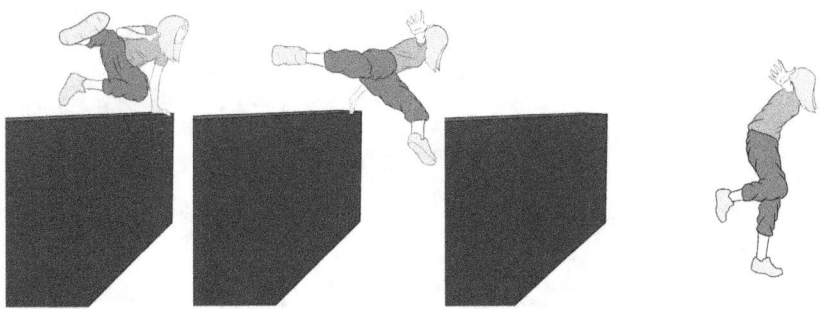

Note: If you want to exit in a direction other than straight ahead, try to face your chest in the direction you want to go and use your hand on the wall as a pivot point.

Related Chapters:

- Safety Vault
- Lazy Vault

TURN VAULT

The turn vault can be used to pass over a rail, wall, fence, ledge, etc. in a swift and safe manner. Besides passing over as usual, another common use of the turn vault is to cat-hang (or just hang) over the other side of an obstacle before dropping down.

It's a good idea to learn the safety vault before attempting the turn vault. This will give you a basic understanding of the body mechanics needed to get over an obstacle and help to build your confidence.

When first learning the turn vault, do it over a rail rather than a wall. If you're worried about clearing the height, you can first try it at the end of the rail so your legs can just come around the end if needed.

Start with a rail about waist height.

Place your hands on the rail a comfortable distance apart (shoulder-width is usually good), with one hand facing up and the other facing down. Your legs will go in the direction of the hand facing down, which is the hand you will take off the rail.

Squat back so your arms are almost straight, and then push up with your legs while pulling with your arms to arc up and over the rail. Your legs should swing around to the side.

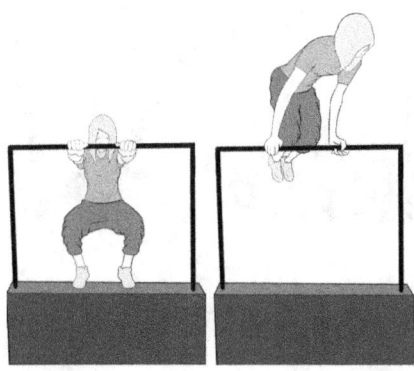

Your chest should come over the bar first. As your legs come over the bar, release your hand so you can complete the 180° spin.

Once you're on the other side place, your hand back on the bar in an overhand position, at about the same distance as it was originally. As you're doing this, you also want to be looking at where to place your feet.

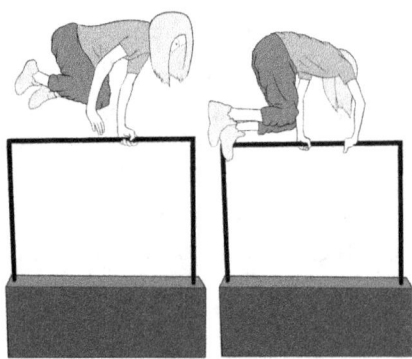

As you come down to land, lean back a little and place your feet on the target. Leaning back allows the energy to get pushed through your feet, which will give you a good grip.

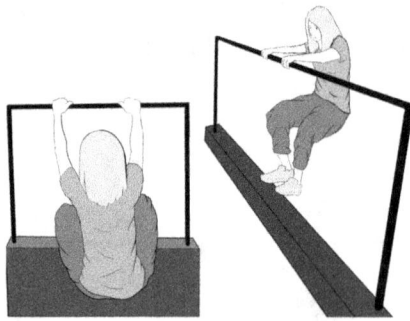

Don't worry if you can't get your hand and foot in the right place on the other side right away. Just keep practicing.

Once you can do the turn vault on a rail smoothly, you can progress to using a wall/ledge. You'll need to adjust your hand positioning since you can't grab under a wall. Somewhere close to 90° to the side is good.

Come over in the usual way, but use less speed, so you can hold yourself up on the other side.

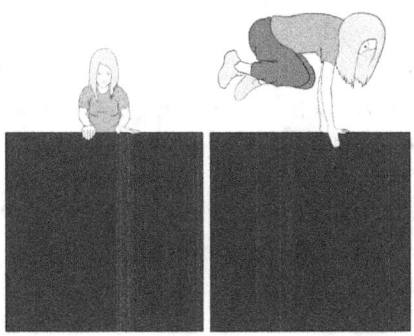

Once you're stable, you can drop down into a cat-hang or do whatever else you want.

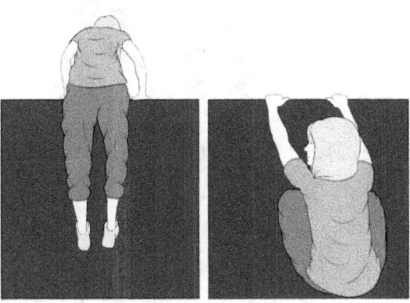

Once you're confident/have built enough strength, you can use more speed and go straight into a cat-hang.

Related Chapters:

- Safety Vault

REVERSE SAFETY VAULT

The reverse safety vault (a.k.a. reverse step vault) is a good progression technique to use to work up to the reverse vault, but it also has a lot of practical uses in its own right.

If you're backed up against an obstacle, you can use the reverse safety vault to pass over it without having to turn to face it. Then you can either land to face your aggressor or land facing away so you can run. You can also use it to back out of numerous types of forward-facing vaults if you see danger on the other side.

Stand with your back to the obstacle and place your right hand on it, fingers facing forward. Hop up onto it, with your left foot making contact.

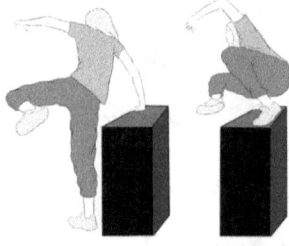

Push off with your left foot so that you turn to your left and land on the other side, facing away from the obstacle. Land on your right foot first.

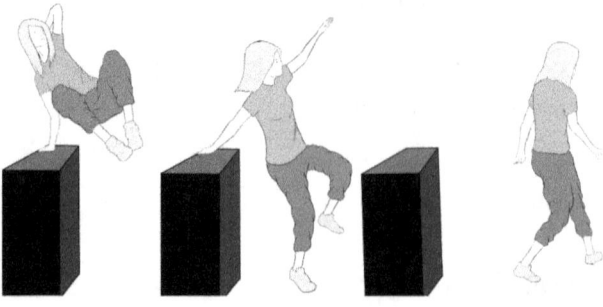

Eventually you want to be able to do this smoothly, without having to look at your foot as you come up onto the obstacle.

Practice it so you stay facing the same way as well. Instead of pushing off with your left foot to spin, just place your right foot onto the ground.

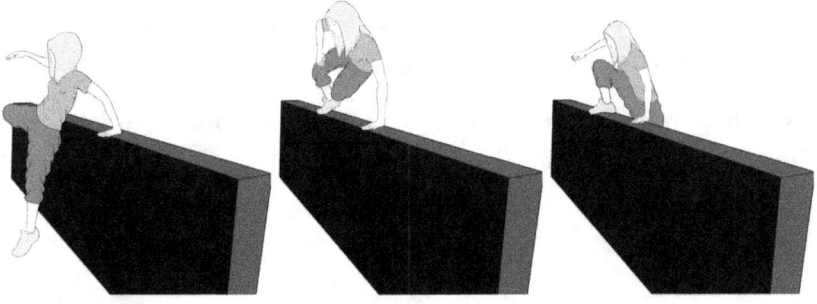

Related Chapters:

- Reverse Vault

LAZY VAULT

The lazy vault is useful when approaching a small to medium-sized obstacle at an angle other than straight on, and no matter what speed your approach is.

It can be used when coming in and out on a similar angle, and it can also be adapted to exit on a different angle.

Assuming you are approaching the obstacle from your left, your limbs should go over the wall in this order:

1. Left hand.
2. Left leg.
3. Right leg.
4. Right hand.

This first progression step will help you to get the mechanics of the technique.

Approach the wall on a diagonal and place your left hand (#1) on it as you jump up. Your left leg (#2) should come through, so that you land on the wall with your right foot (#3).

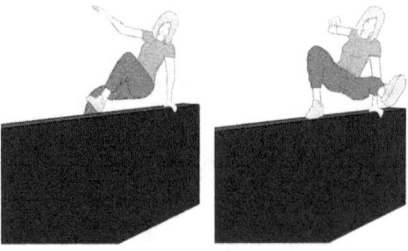

Drop down to the ground, landing on your left foot first (#2), and then continue to run.

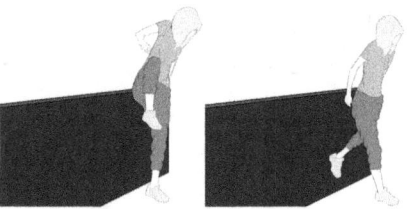

Here it is approaching from the opposite side. Your right hand is #1.

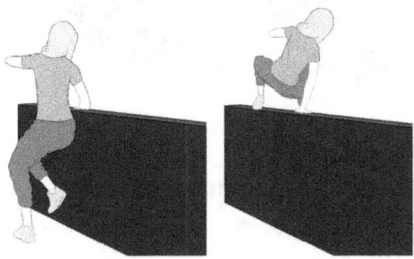

Once you're ready, you can learn the actual lazy vault, which means you will not place your #3 foot on the wall.

Kick your legs up over the wall and bring your hips up.

As you go over, your #4 hand should replace your #2 hand on the obstacle.

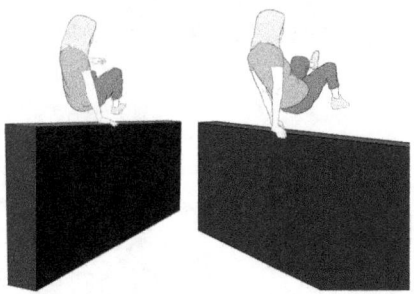

Use your #4 hand to help push your hips away from the obstacle so you can continue running.

A "proper" lazy vault is one in which you approach on an angle and exit along the same path. Ensure your limbs go over in the right order and that you land/run out on #2.

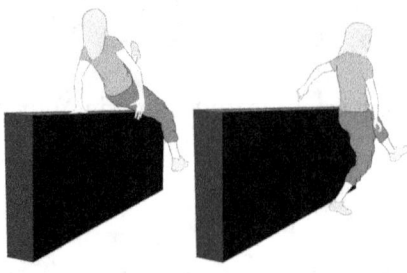

If you want to exit on a different angle, just turn your hips in the direction you want to go while you're still in the air.

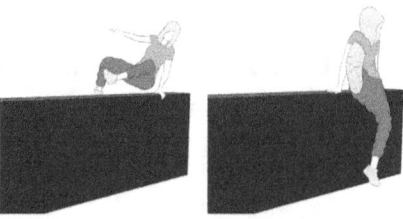

If you are exiting on a different angle unintentionally, it may be because you're forgetting to put your #4 hand down.

KONG VAULT

The kong vault (also known as the cat pass, monkey vault, kong leap, etc.) is useful for vaulting longer or higher obstacles. It's a bit more difficult than the previous vaults explained in this book, but is worth the practice because it's extremely useful.

Start on something wide enough to land on but not too high, like a picnic table, and small enough to vault over (eventually).

This first progression exercise is helpful in getting over the fear of hitting your toes on the obstacle.

Stand at one end of the obstacle and place your palms flat on it a little more than shoulder-width apart, with your fingers facing forwards.

Use your arms to support you as you jump up onto the obstacle, landing with your feet between your hands. Move your hands away as needed.

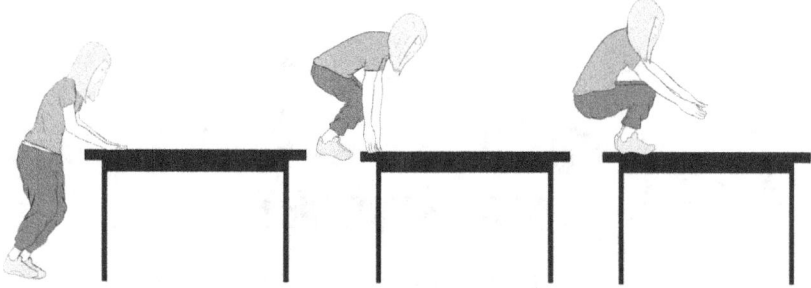

Repeat this exercise until you're comfortable with the mechanics.

When you're ready, try to land further and further forward with your feet by pushing the obstacle back underneath you. The more you push, the further you can go.

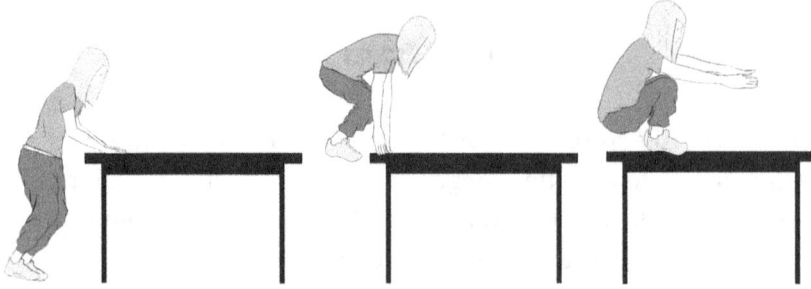

Next try starting with some distance between you and the obstacle. Take a one- or two-step run-up, then do the same as before.

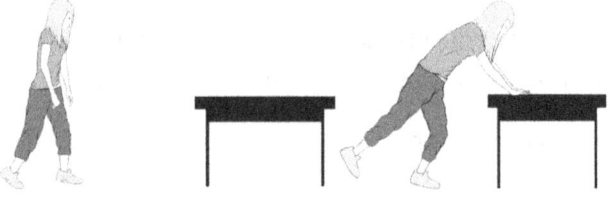

Let the momentum help you to get further onto the obstacle.

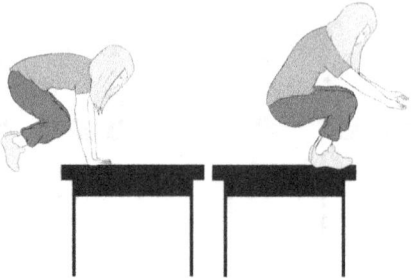

To get even further, you can run up with a bit more momentum, using one of two take-offs depending on the type of obstacle.

First, try the two-foot punch take off, which most people find easier. It will redirect momentum up, which makes it better for high obstacles.

Start further away from the obstacle than you have been. Run up and hop on one foot.

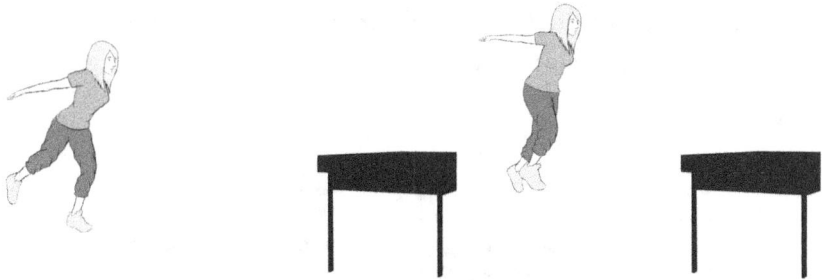

Land on both feet together, then use the momentum to go into a dive onto the obstacle before completing the vault as normal.

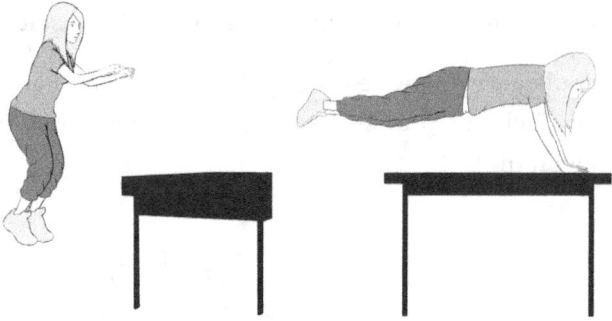

You will need practice to learn where a good distance is for you to land back from the obstacle.

Next, try the split-foot take-off. This take-off has more forward momentum than the two-foot punch take-off, which makes it better for longer obstacles.

Start at about the same distance as you did for the two-foot punch take off. Run up and hop on one foot, then land on the opposite one.

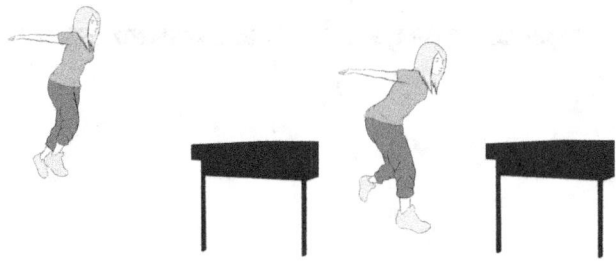

Take another quick step then push up with both feet to go into the dive. Complete the vault as before.

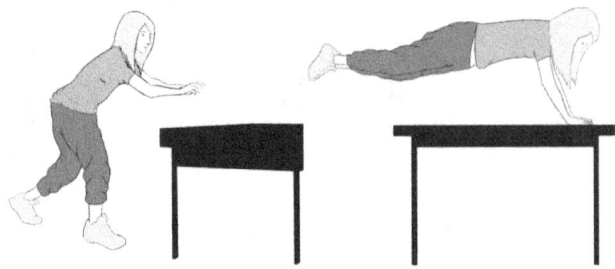

Try to get further and further, until you can clear the obstacle.

To get more distance, increase your approach speed and use the split-foot take-off. Kick out your feet to raise your hips, which will help stretch out your dive.

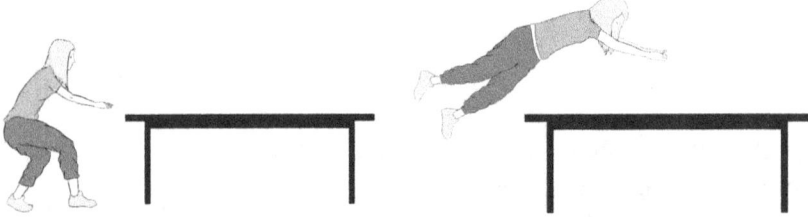

Spot where you want your hands to land, and then push up and forward as your arms make contact.

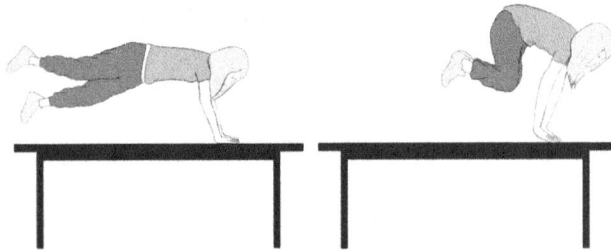

Land on two feet to begin with, and then progress into landing in a one-two motion so you can resume running.

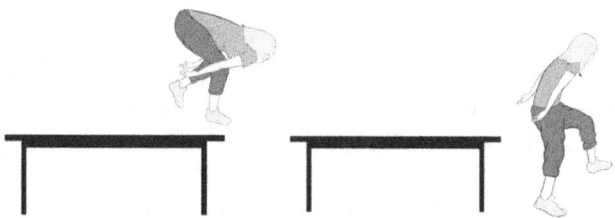

Once you are comfortable, try the kong vault on higher and/or longer obstacles using the appropriate take-off—the two-foot punch for higher ones and the split foot for longer ones.

REVERSE VAULT

The reverse vault is useful when you have a lot of momentum but not enough space to dive or swing your leg. This may be because two obstacles are very close together, or because someone has swung you with your back towards an obstacle.

There are two good ways to learn the reverse vault.

The first is to get faster and faster at the reverse safety vault. The more you do it, the less you'll need to put the weight on your foot, until eventually you will be able to get all the way over the obstacle and land on the other side in a standard reverse vault.

The second way is to build up from side sapiens. For detailed instructions on how to do side sapiens, see the section on warm-ups and conditioning.

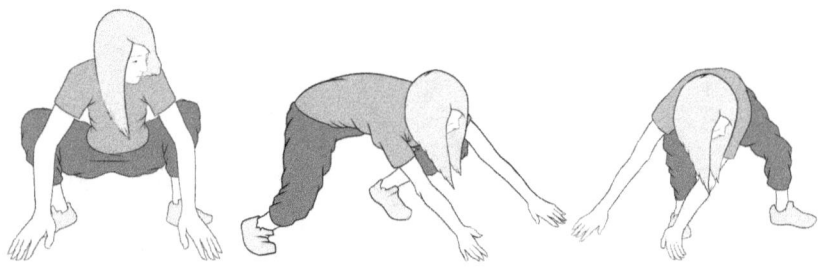

Once you are comfortable with side sapiens, try the following twisting variation of it. Face forward, and then place your hands as if doing side sapiens, but at a 90° angle.

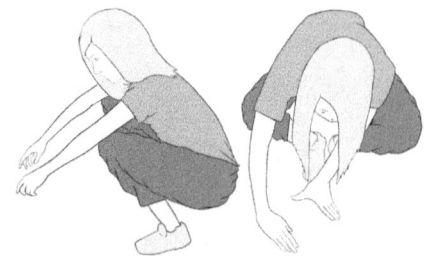

Use your arms to support your weight as you turn in a circle, until you're facing forward again.

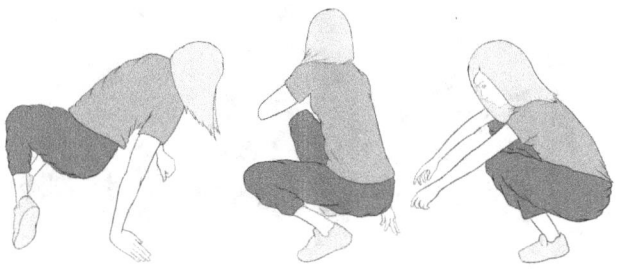

This twisting motion variation of side sapiens can also be adapted to save you if you're sitting on something and fall (or are pushed) backwards.

The next progression is to do side sapiens over an obstacle.

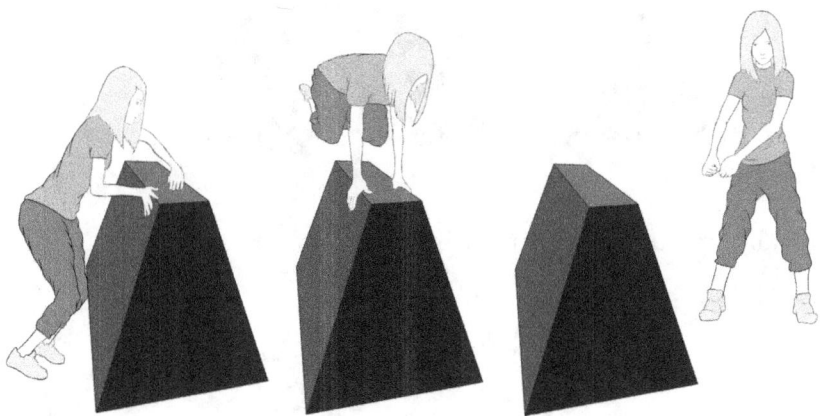

When you are ready, add a full twist as you come down out of the move.

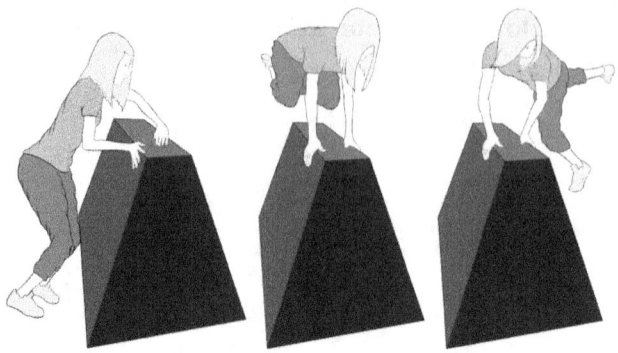

Land on the foot closest to the obstacle first, and keep spinning until you're facing away from it.

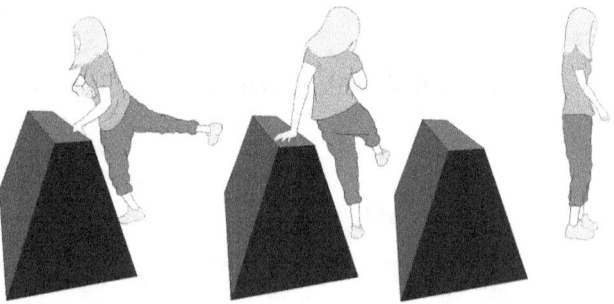

Finally, start the twist from the beginning.

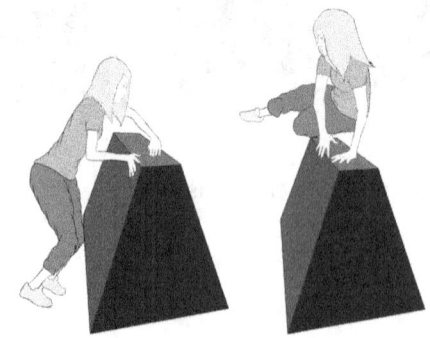

Finish by landing in the same way as before.

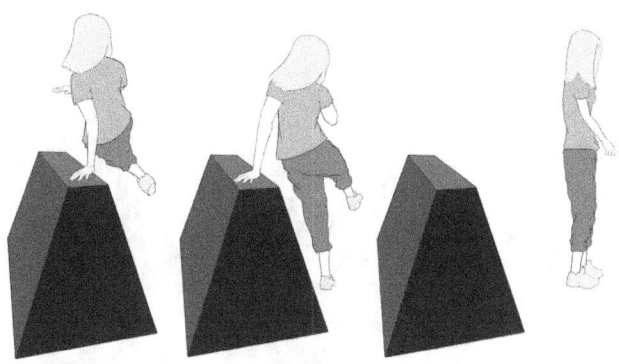

Practice this vault immediately after other vaults when the obstacles are close together or while you're being flung into one.

An opponent grabs you and begins to fling you into an obstacle.

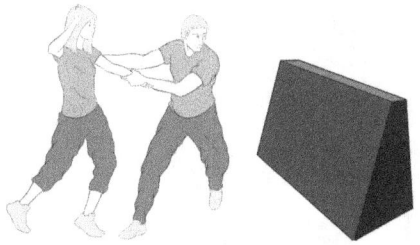

When you are about a step away from the obstacle, start to turn your back to it.

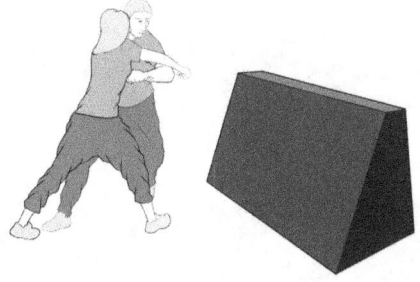

Place your hand on the obstacle first to help gauge distance and direct momentum as you vault over it.

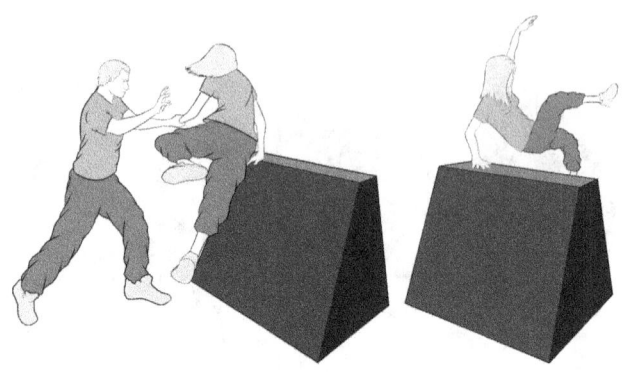

Related Chapters:

- Side Sapiens
- Reverse Safety Vault

WALL TECHNIQUES

This section covers all the techniques that are predominantly associated with walls. They are mostly to do with overcoming obstacles that are too big to vault.

CAT LEAP TO CAT HANG

The cat leap (a.k.a. the arm jump, arm leap, etc.) to cat hang is a commonly used technique in which you jump towards a vertical obstacle (cat leap) and hang off it (cat hang).

The standard cat leap is from a precision or running jump, but other techniques, such as a kong vault or a lache, are also often used.

Once in the cat hang, you can choose to drop down, climb up, cat to cat, etc. The cat hang is also very useful in its own right, since it can be used to lower yourself to the ground. You can do a turn vault to cat hang and then drop down.

When first learning the cat leap to cat hang, start from a stationary position fairly close to the obstacle.

As you jump toward the obstacle, lean back a little and bring your feet and hands out in front of you. Arc into your landing and connect with the obstacle feet-first so that your feet can absorb the impact.

Keep a little space between your feet as you land, so that if you fall back you have more control.

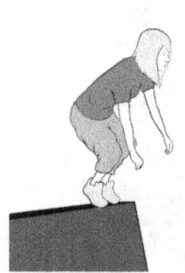 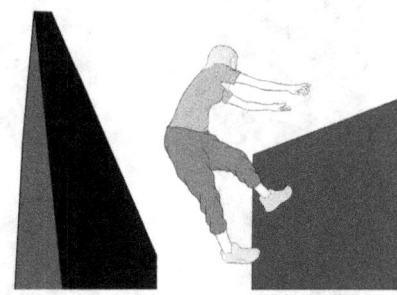

If it is a low obstacle, avoid landing too high on it otherwise you will find it harder to grab the top.

Note: It is very important to connect with the obstacle feet-first. If you don't, you'll probably just slam into it.

Once you have grabbed onto the top of the obstacle, you can straighten your arms so you are "crouching" against the wall. This is the cat hang. From here, you can drop down or climb up.

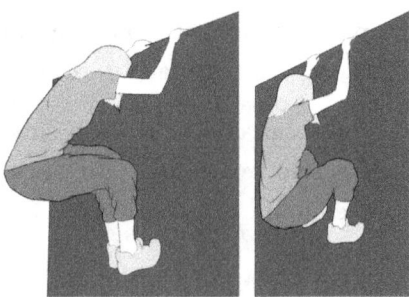

If dropping down, kick away from the obstacle a little bit and turn away from it on your way down. Land with a safety tap or roll.

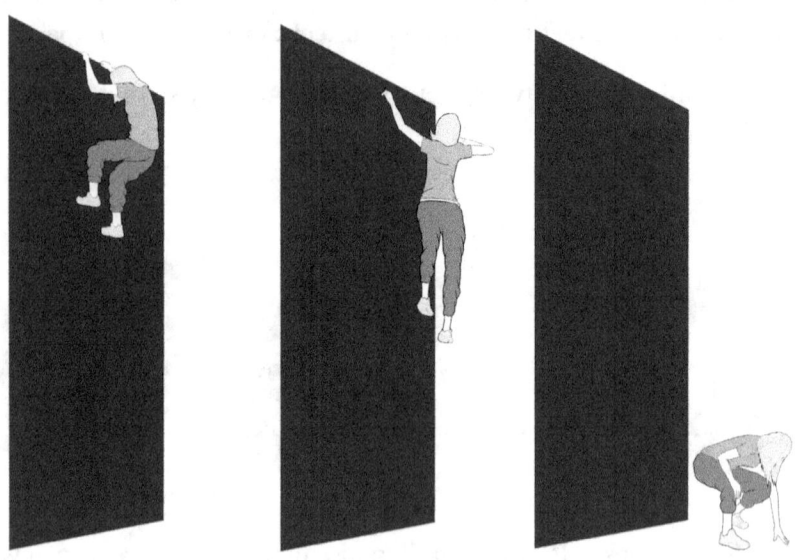

Practice with different heights, distances, etc., so you get used adjusting your jump in different circumstances.

Related Chapters:

- Safety Tap
- Turn Vault
- Kong Vault
- Cat to Cat
- Lache
- Wall Climb-up
- Safety Rolls

CAT TO CAT

The cat to cat is when you leap from one cat hang to another one on an opposing obstacle.

Before learning the cat to cat, you need to know the cat hang.

Find two obstacles that directly face one another. This makes it easier to learn to begin with.

Go into a cat hang on the first obstacle.

Turn you head to spot where you're going to land, and push off with one of your legs as you let go with your hands.

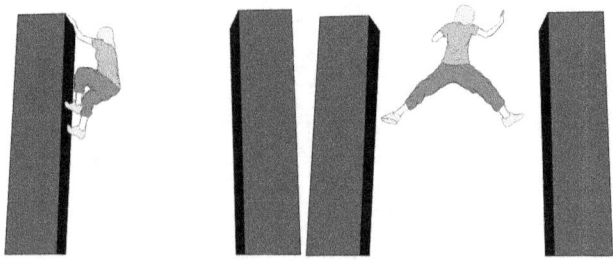

Immediately turn to face the second obstacle and reach out with your other leg (the opposite of the one you pushed off with) so it's ready to absorb the impact before you take a grip with your hands to land in a cat hang.

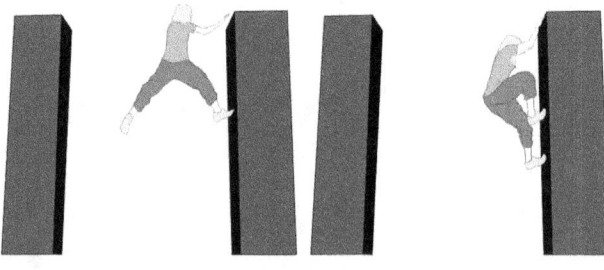

Once you're confident, practice with different angles, heights, cat to precision, cat to crane, cat to lache, etc.

In all cases, the main thing is to be aware of is how your feet and hands hit the wall.

When you're going from low to high, you want to get a lot of pressure into the wall, so that your feet don't slip as you push your body up.

When you're going from high to low, make sure that you still get your feet out in front of you and that you're lowering yourself into the landing with your chest back. This will keep you from hitting your face.

Related Chapters:

- Lache
- Precision Jumping
- Crane Landing

TIC-TAC

A tic-tac is when you push your foot off an obstacle on an angle. It's a fairly simple technique that can be used to help you clear gaps, leap over obstacles, gain height, or quickly redirect your momentum.

A horizontal wall run is a progression of the tic-tac in which you take multiple steps along the wall, as opposed to just one.

To begin with, just get used to how the obstacle feels under your foot. Walk up to the obstacle, place your foot on it, and then push off in a slight upward manner so you arc back onto the ground. Land on the foot opposite the one you pushed off with first and then continue to walk away.

You can either focus your tic-tac on pushing away from the obstacle or pushing along it, so experiment with both by facing your chest and shoulders towards your destination.

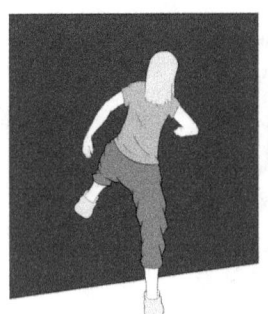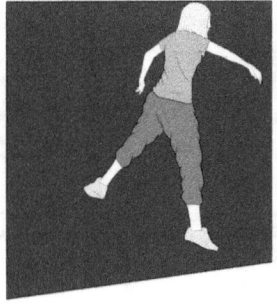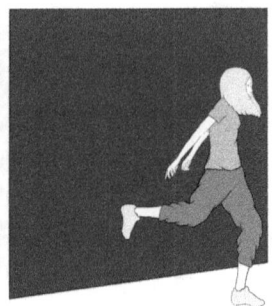

Next, start to add some momentum and try to get increasing distance and/or height.

The more momentum you have, the harder you can push off the wall and the higher and/or farther you will be able to get. As well, the higher you place your foot on the obstacle, the more lift and distance you will achieve.

Once you're confident, you can start doing it over objects.

Concentrate on your foot placement so you can get enough leverage off the wall to clear the object.

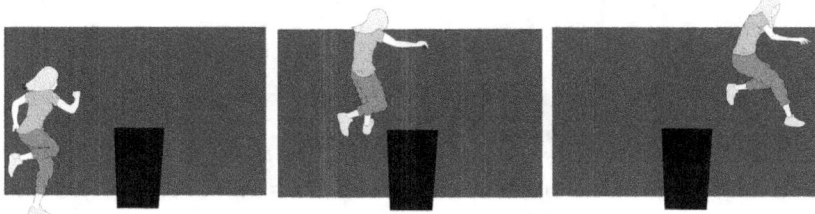

Then try with multiple steps. This is where the tic-tac turns into the horizontal wall run.

Approach at a smaller angle between you and the wall. First try with two steps, then three or more.

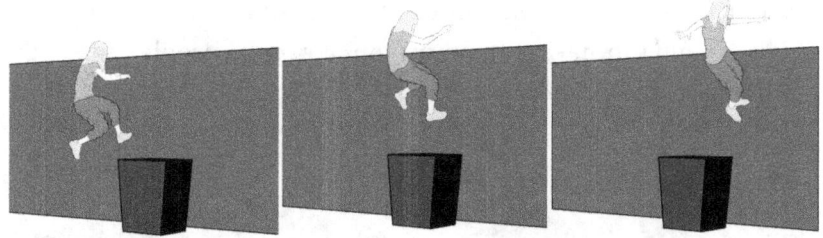

The tic-tac can also be used to help you get over higher obstacles.

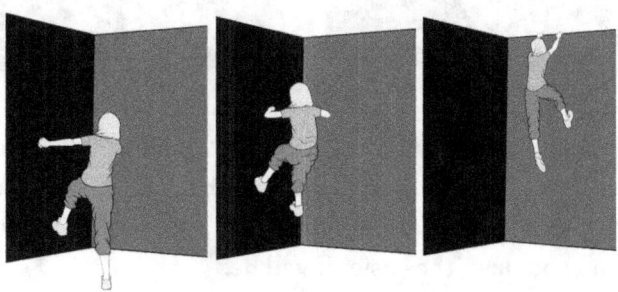

WALL CLIMB-UP

The wall climb-up is used to pull yourself from a hanging position up onto a wall quickly and efficiently.

When you're first learning, it will help to use the momentum from a cat leap or wall run to help get up the wall. Eventually, you'll want to be able to do it from a static hang.

Start on a wall you can easily cat leap to cat hang to, so that you can get the most out of your momentum.

As soon as you have a grip on the obstacle, use your feet to push your hips back as you pull up and in with your arms. Push your feet into the obstacle, not down. Try to straighten your highest leg.

Your leg push and arm pull should be one smooth motion. The aim is to get your chest above the top of the obstacle.

As your chest comes over, you need to transition from having your hands hanging to having them on top. For most people, this is the hardest part of the climb-up.

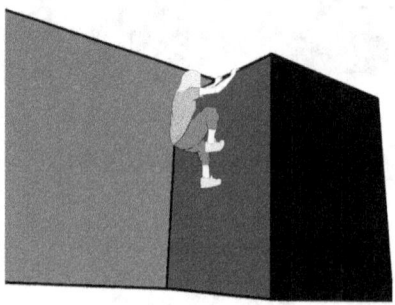 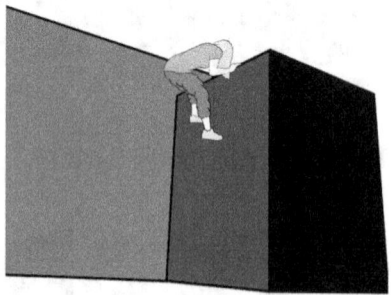

Using the momentum from the push/pull, quickly take the weight off your hands and pop them on top of the obstacle, so that your palms are on it. The more you can push against the obstacle and the more momentum you have, the easier it will be.

When you're first learning, you can do the transition one arm at a time and then progress to doing them together when you're ready.

Once your hands are on top, push up. Keep your chest forward so you don't fall back. To stand on the obstacle, use one of your feet to kick out a little.

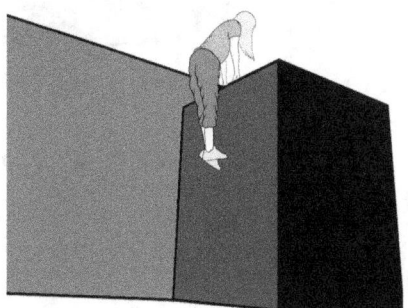 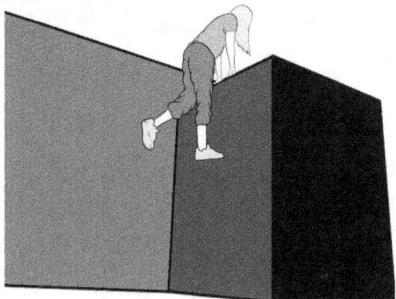

Bring your other foot up on top. Avoid using your elbows and knees to help you.

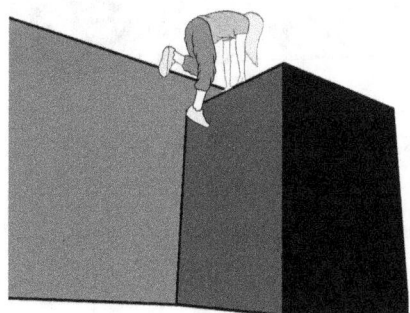 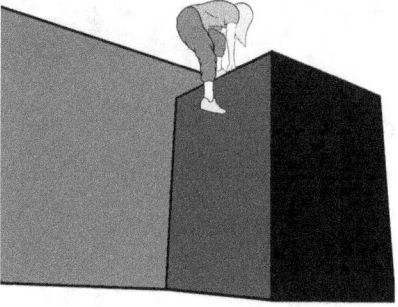

Alternatively, you can do the wall pop-up to stand.

Once you can do the wall climb-up, try doing it from a static hang. Push your body against the obstacle a little to help pop your hips back.

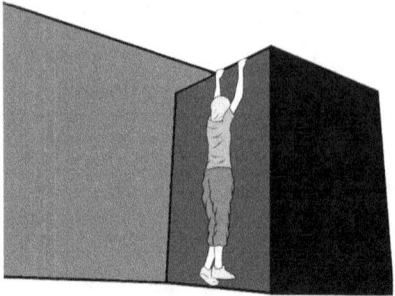 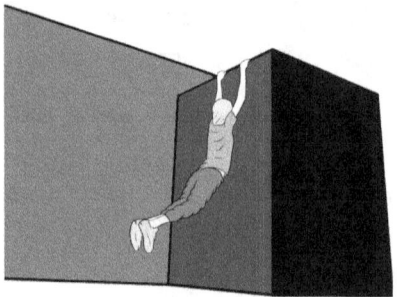

As your legs swing back in, place one foot on the wall and then get your other leg as high as possible so you can transition into the wall climb-up.

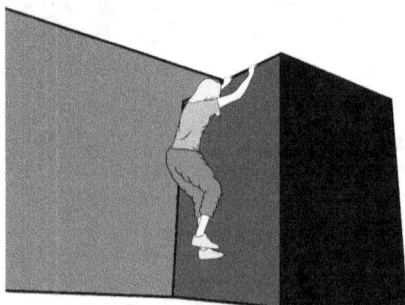 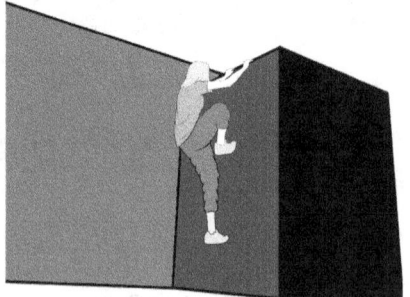

Correct technique is what will get you on top of an obstacle, but having more strength will make it easier, especially when you're doing it from a static hang. Some useful exercises to help build strength are:

- **Dips.** With your hands in front of your chest to mimic the climb-up, as opposed to being out to your sides.
- **Pull ups.** Standard pull-ups. Not to be confused with chin-ups.
- **Reverse climb-ups.** Start from on top of the wall and slowly lower yourself down by reversing the climb-up action.
- **Super-burpees.** The ultimate all-round conditioning exercise.

- **Traversing.** Hang off an obstacle and traverse around it.

Eventually, you can progress to a one-armed wall climb-up from a static hang.

Related Chapters:

- Pull-ups
- Cat Leap to Cat Hang
- Wall Pop-up

VERTICAL WALL RUN

Use the vertical wall run to get up tall obstacles.

To practice the vertical wall run, you can use any obstacle that is tall enough. You don't have to be able to reach the top to practice, but if you can, it means you can also practice your wall climb (or other techniques) at the same time. Small wall runs may also be used as part of a wall pop-up.

Initially, you will have to get familiar with your steps so you have the right pacing when approaching the obstacle. After a while, this will become intuitive.

Find a spot where you're comfortable with your leg resting on the obstacle at about hip height. It shouldn't be so close you're pushing in or so far away where you're stretching to reach.

Once you've found that space, you can start to get comfortable with setting a foot on the obstacle and jumping off it. Don't worry about gaining height yet.

Use your strong leg against the obstacle first, as that's the one that's going to have the most impact. Eventually, you'll want to practice on both sides.

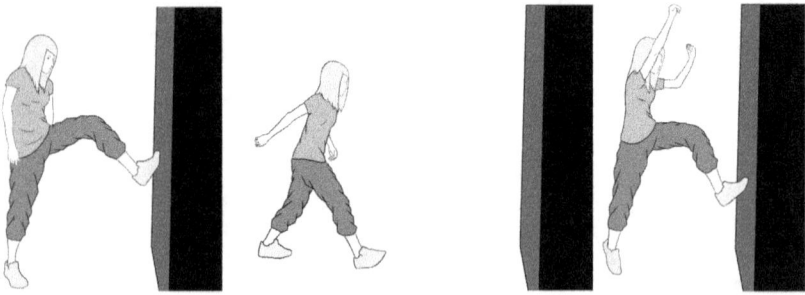

As your foot hits the obstacle, push into it in an upward motion. The aim is to get your center of gravity to go up. Do not apply too much downward pressure, as it will cause you to slip. Run into the obstacle and bounce up off it.

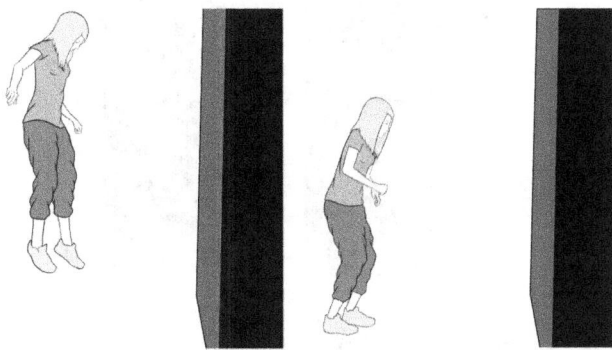

Once you're comfortable add some speed so you can get more height. Don't go too fast too soon, or you might just slam into the obstacle.

Jump and plant your foot as high as you can, then quickly kick off. If you're too slow to kick off, you will lose power.

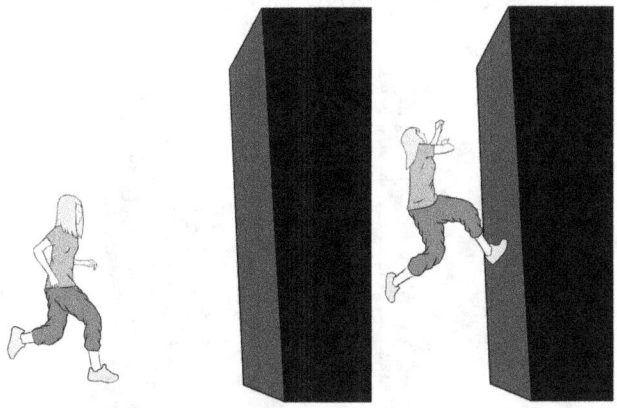

If the obstacle is small, you can try grabbing onto the edge. If not, just touch it at as high a point as you can, keeping in mind that the higher you go, the longer the drop back down will be.

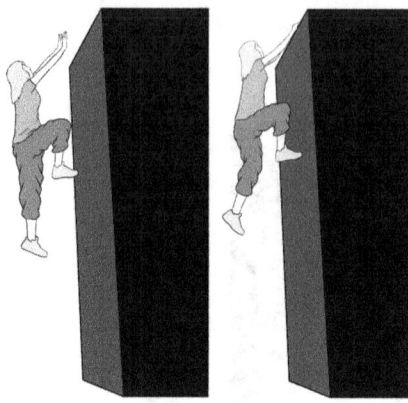

After some practice, you'll be able to recognize how to react according to the obstacle, varying your approach speed, when to jump, how high to plant your foot, etc., accordingly.

Throwing your arms up will give you more reach, as will leading with one arm.

Leaving your hand on the obstacle can be useful to give you a little extra push up, as well as to prevent yourself from slamming into it.

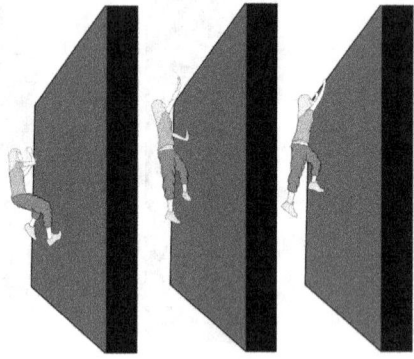

Related Chapters:

- Wall Pop-up

WALL POP-UP

The wall pop-up is used to quickly get over or on top of obstacles that are too high to vault over, but low enough that you don't feel the need to use the wall climb-up.

It can also be used in conjunction with the wall climb. Once you're in the "up" position of the wall climb, use the pop vault to get on top of the wall.

When you're first learning the wall pop-up, do it on an obstacle that's just a little difficult for you to kong vault over.

The first progression for the wall pop-up is to do it with a crane landing.

Do a vertical wall run, but because the obstacle is low, instead of having to hang off it just use your arms give you a little bit of a boost up and then land in a crane landing. A powerful kick off the wall is essential.

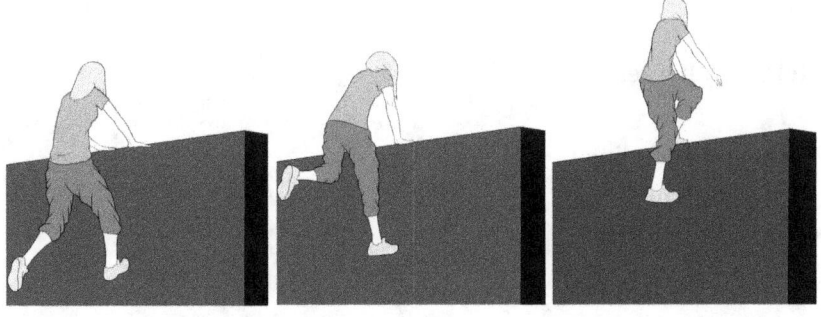

Once you can do that, try bringing both feet up to the side.

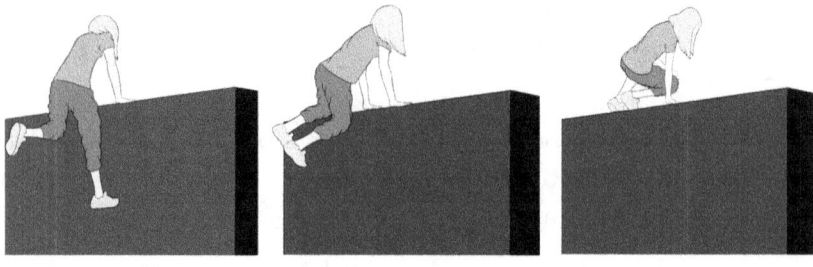

Finally, you can do the full wall pop-up by bringing both your feet up to land on top of the obstacle. The movement is like that used in a kong vault.

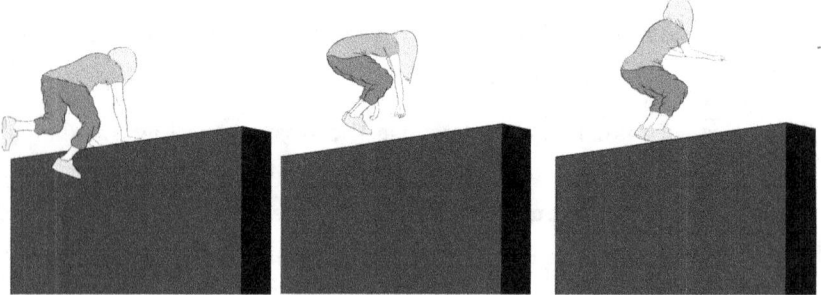

Related Chapters:

- Crane Landing
- Kong Vault
- Wall Climb-up
- Vertical Wall Run

CORNER WALL RUN

The corner wall run is when you use two walls in a corner to gain extra height. It's like doing a tic-tac off one wall to gain height on the second wall, which you then continue to "run" up. Before attempting the corner wall run, you should be proficient with the vertical wall run and the tic-tac.

First, get comfortable with doing the tic-tac off one wall and then pushing off the other. You'll need to be quick to react with your feet. Decide which wall you want to hit first. If it's on your left side, you'll use your left foot to come into it, and if it's on your right side, you'll use your right foot to come into it.

Come in at about a 45° angle and place your foot at about hip level to tic-tac from the first wall into the second.

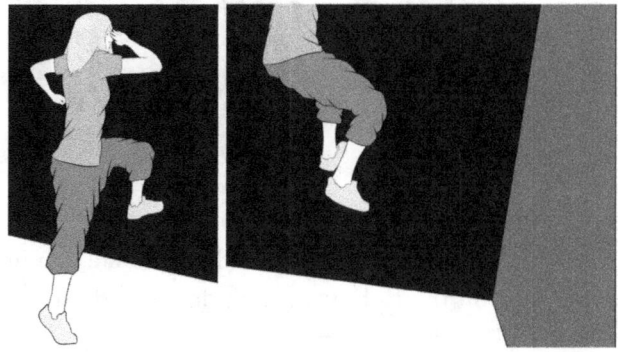

Use your other foot to push back on the second wall (again at about hip level) and then come down to land using a safety tap.

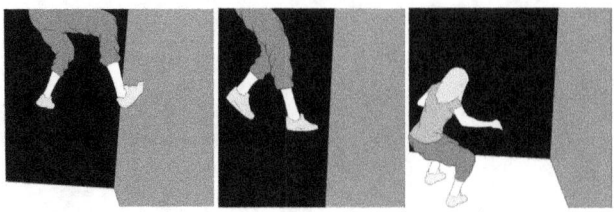

Your arms/hands can help you push on the wall or you can throw them up for more vertical momentum. Test the angle at which you come in on the first wall so you can get the best push off it.

Continue to practice this gradually, adding more speed so you can get more height. Apply basic wall-run techniques for more vertical lift.

When you're ready, add in the wall run on the second wall so you can reach the top of the obstacle. Foot placement and explosiveness are the keys. You need lots of power and the right angle into the first tic-tac so you can get more momentum off the second step to continue the wall run.

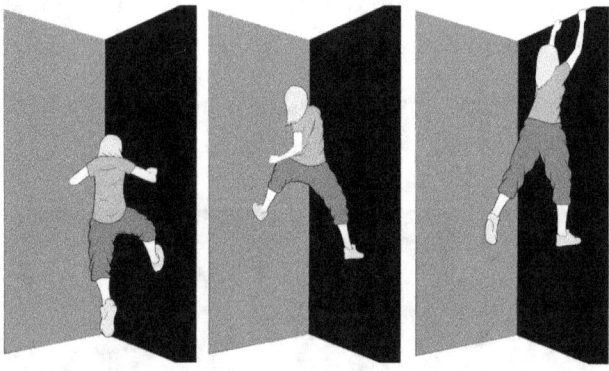

The above pictures show moving from the left wall to the right and then back to the left to grab the top of the obstacle. An alternative would be to tic-tac off the right wall then do a standard vertical wall run up the left wall to grab the top.

Related Chapters:

- Safety Tap
- Tic-Tac
- Vertical Wall Run

BAR TECHNIQUES

This section covers techniques that are predominantly associated with bars and that have not been covered in previous sections.

STRAIGHT UNDERBAR

The straight underbar allows you to smoothly pass under and/or between bars or other obstacles, like ledges.

When you're first learning the straight underbar, you want to progress very slowly. If you go too fast too soon, you'll probably end up getting injured.

Find an obstacle with a good-sized gap to pass though. Going from low to high will be easier than going from high to low, as it will give you more control with your feet on the other side.

When doing the underbar, let your feet lead your body and your hands grab the obstacle to help control your body as you go through.

Stand next to the bar and stick one leg through, then the other.

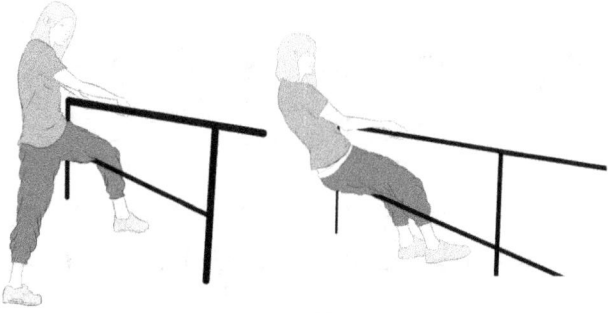

Slowly work your body through. Use this slow speed to become familiar with the distance between your body parts and the obstacle as you go through.

Give extra attention to your back and head, as they are most likely to hit. Be very careful you don't hit your head.

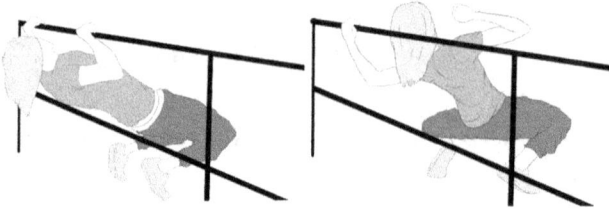

Once you're comfortable, gradually get faster. Try to get straighter as well, rather than coming in side on.

Lead with your feet, lean back a little, and reach forward to grab the bar with your hands so you can pull yourself through.

Lie back as you pull, so your upper torso and head can pass through. Direct your legs upwards.

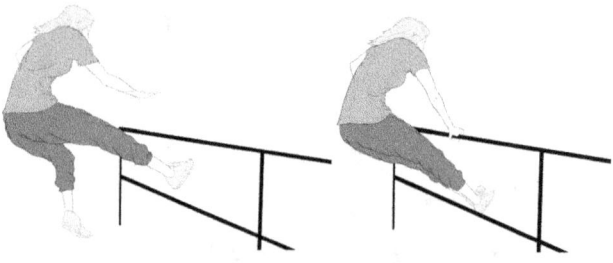

You can swing your legs slightly to the side if needed to avoid hitting your knees or shins.

Next, try different variations. Practice high to low, low to high, smaller gaps, more speed, coming from the side, gap jump to underbar, etc.

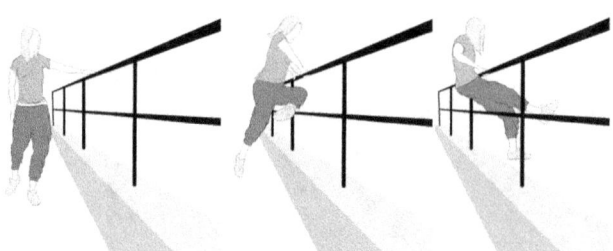

When you're doing gap jumps to underbars, aim with your feet, similar to the way you would with a precision jump. Aim them through the gap, so the rest of your body will follow along the same path.

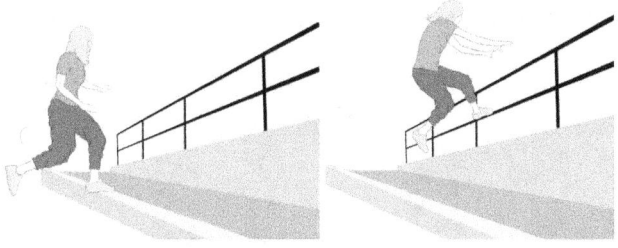

Don't lean back too much, and as soon as you grab the bar, control the way the rest of your body comes through.

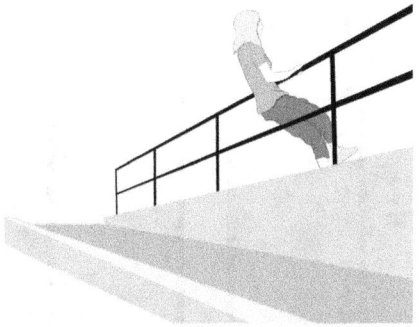

Note: When you're going under (not between) something about chest to head height, doing the underbar is usually unnecessary, but you should still use your hand on the obstacle above you as a guide so that you don't hit your head.

LACHE

The lache is used to swing off a bar (or branch, or anything else you can swing from) and then land in precision, crane, or cat position, or grab onto another bar (lache to lache).

Knowing how to lache properly will allow you to propel yourself a much greater distance from the bar.

The Swing

The most important part of every lache is swinging. Don't just try to swing with your legs. You need to use your shoulders, chest, torso, etc.

Start in a stationary hang on the bar. Get your feet behind you and curve your spine backwards.

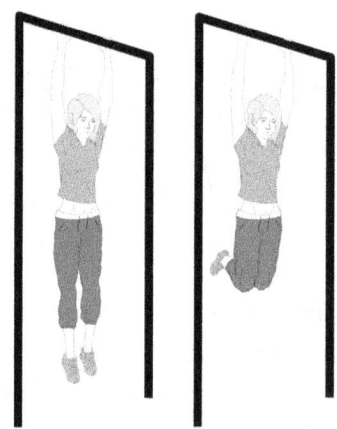

Bend your knees to your chest and then push your feet out and up. Keep your arms straight. This is a flowing movement done in an explosive manner.

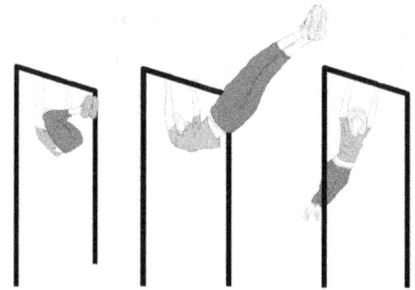

Lache to Precision

Once you have the correct swing technique, you can attempt the lache to precision. If you don't know how to precision jump yet, learn that first.

As with any precision jump, you need to know where you want to land. Choose any spot (line, crack, etc.) on the ground that you're confident you can reach.

You also need to be able to see that landing spot as you release your hands. To do this, you need to release your hands one at a time.

As your body goes forward, release one of your hands and keep it in front of your eyes. When you gain enough speed, release your second hand and keep your eyes on the line that you're going to land on.

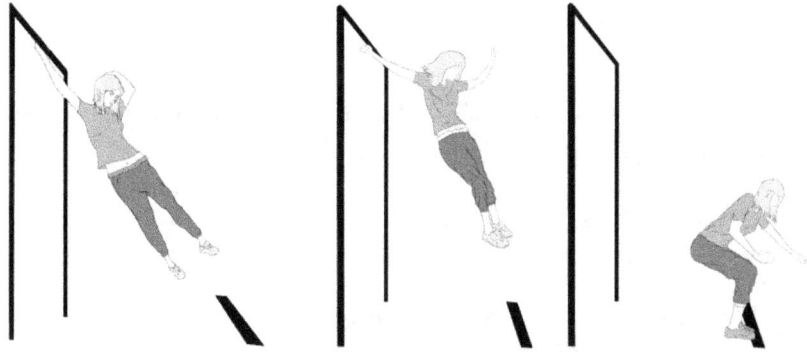

This arm-releasing technique stays the same no matter how far you want to go or what type of lache you're doing. Always release one hand first, then the other.

To precision further, you just need to get more momentum in the swing.

Lache to Lache

For the lache to lache, instead of focusing on a landing point you need to focus on the next bar you'll grab onto.

To do continuous lache to lache, you need to grab the next bar with your legs behind you, so that you maintain enough speed for the next swing.

Start to swing and release your first hand as your legs go in front of you. As you release your second hand, swing your legs behind you. Then catch the bar.

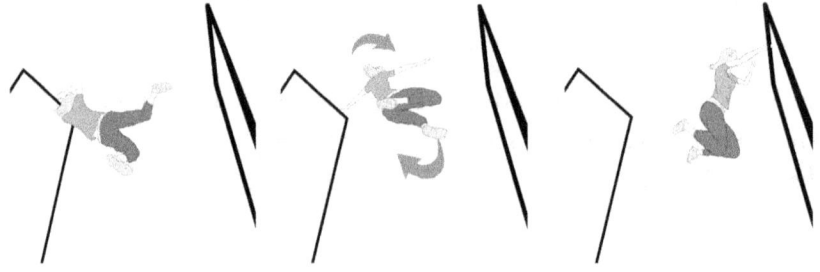

Swing your legs forward again and then repeat the movement, lache to lache to lache.

Lache to Cat Leap

The lache to cat leap is a combination of the lache to precision and the lache to lache. It's lache to precision because you have to land on the wall with your legs, and it's lache to lache because you'll have to grab something with your arms.

If you don't know how to cat leap to cat hang yet, learn that first.

The arm release is the same. Let go with one hand first, then the other. Keep your legs in front of you the whole time, so you can absorb the impact as you land in cat.

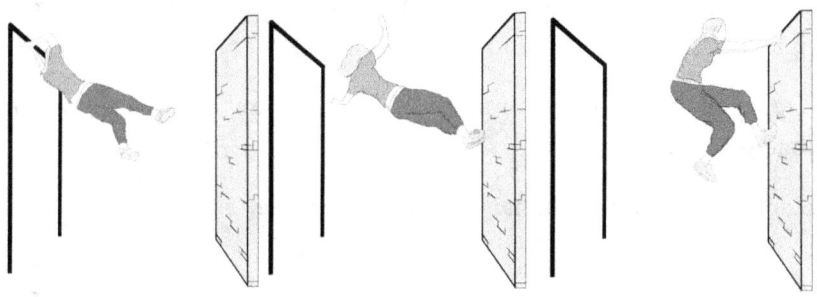

Related Chapters:

- Cat Leap to Cat Hang
- Precision Jumping

MONKEY TRAVERSE

The monkey traverse (a.k.a. the sloth shimmy) is used to get across long-distance obstacles that you can hang off. It is safer than cat-walking on the bar, and works on rope too.

Hang below the obstacle, suspended by your hands and with both feet crossed over the rope. Your left hand should be in front of your right hand and your right foot should be in front of your left foot.

Keep a slight bend in your arms and engage your core for the whole time you're are traversing.

Start to move your right hand in front of your left hand.

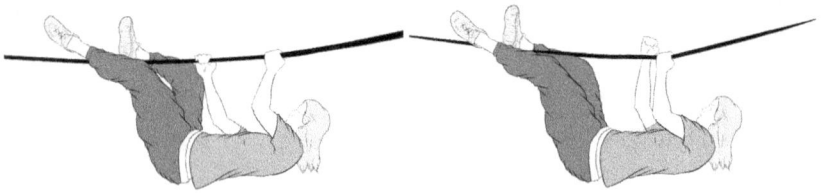

As you take a grip with your right hand, move your left foot in front of your right. Do not slide your feet. Lift them. This will prevent friction burns.

Ensure your feet land ahead of each other and not on top; otherwise, you'll get tangled up.

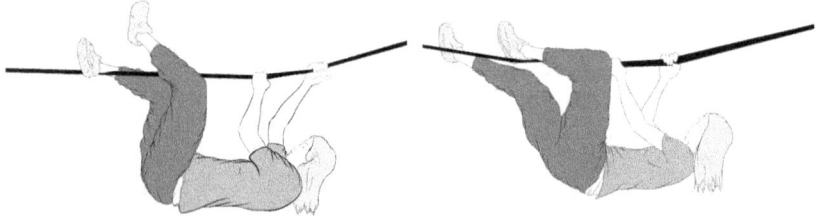

Continue this motion.

MUSCLE-UPS

Muscle-ups are used to get on top of higher obstacles, like overhanging ledges, in cases where a wall climb-up cannot be used.

You'll need to be proficient at the wall climb-up before attempting the muscle-up, for both technique and conditioning reasons.

The muscle-up is quite a physically demanding exercise. Progressing gradually is the key to success.

Start with the hanging knee to elbow leg raise.

Hang off the bar and pull yourself up slightly to retract your shoulder blades. This will help keep you stable while you're doing the exercise.

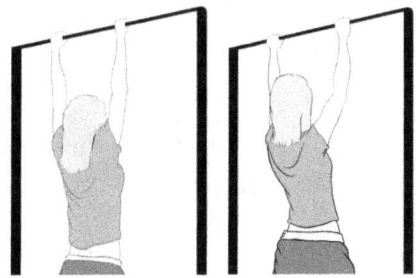

Keep your core tight and swing forward a little bit. As your body starts to swing back thrust your knees to your chest.

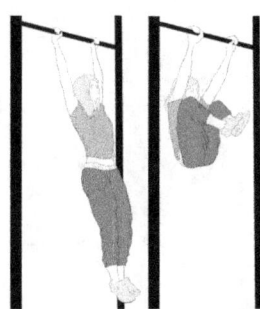

Next, you need to learn how to use the momentum from the hanging knee to elbow raise to pull yourself over the bar.

Start the hanging knee to elbow leg raise as normal. At the height of your back swing, pull yourself forward and thrust your knees to your chest, while allowing your wrists to rotate over the bar. The wrist movement is very important.

It will help if you have access to a lower bar to practice the movement. If not, then just keep it in mind when doing the muscle-up.

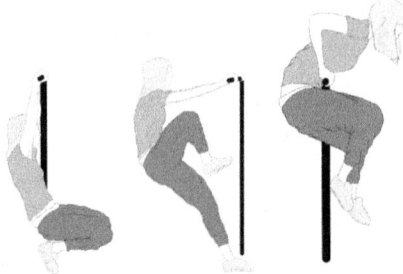

Now you can put everything together to do the muscle-up. It's important to use everything you've learned so far. Remember to keep your core tight.

In addition to retracting your shoulder blades, pull your arms forward a little bit when pulling yourself over the bar.

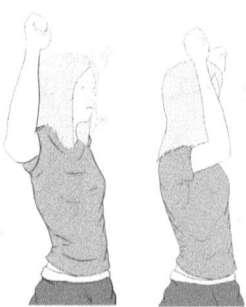

You can use some chalk to get extra grip, although you probably won't have this luxury in real-life scenarios.

Get some momentum, and then thrust your knees to your chest.

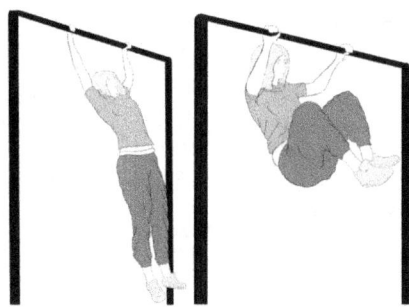

As you do so, ensure your wrists are loosened. At the right moment, pull yourself up over the bar. Push yourself up until your arms are fully extended.

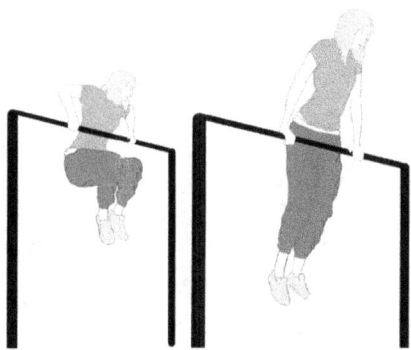

If this was an obstacle, you would bring your foot up and stand, just like in the wall-climb.

If you want to do multiple muscle-ups, you can use the momentum you gain when lowering yourself down to go into the next repetition.

Once you've built more strength, try to do the muscle-up with less and less swing, until you can do it from a dead hang.

You'll also need to practice doing muscle-ups over hanging ledges, where there are no walls for your feet to push against. To do this, you need to adjust your technique a little, since you don't have a bar for your wrist to rotate over. Use the "pop" hand movement you use when doing a wall climb-up.

Related Chapters:

- Wall Climb-up

BOULDERING

Bouldering is the act of climbing without the use of ropes and harnesses.

I haven't met many people who didn't enjoy climbing when they were a child. Trees, rocks, the roof of the family home—I loved to climb them all, and perhaps you did too. The point is that as children, we needed no instruction on how to climb; we just did. That's because climbing is a natural instinct in all of us.

As we get older and stop "practicing," we lose the skills. Luckily, they can be relearned, and in the process we can also learn the best methods to use.

The only intention of this section is to introduce the basic maneuvers and foundational techniques needed for bouldering. The basics are all you really need. Learn and practice them.

Safety note: When bouldering, NEVER climb higher than you would be willing to jump down. It's also wise to use a crash mat.

It is a good idea to learn the safety tap which you can find in the Parkour section of this book.

Related Chapters:

- Safety Tap

BASIC PRINCIPLES

Holds are what you place your feet and hands on when climbing. They are what you "hold" on to.

Climb with Your Legs

Your legs are your main climbing tool. Your arms are primarily for keeping balance. Be sure to:

- Move your feet up the wall first and use your legs to push you up.
- Know where you will place your foot before moving it.
- Place your foot carefully and firmly.
- Use the edges of your feet or the ball of your big toe.
- Press your foot firmly downwards and into the wall.
- Trust that you can stand.

Plan Your Route

Plan your route before you start climbing and at least one move ahead while you're climbing. Adjust your plan as needed as you do.

Climb Smoothly

Remember to:

- Climb smoothly and fluidly. Don't pause between moves.
- Step lightly, and only reach as much as needed to grab the hold.
- Grip only as hard as you need to.
- Breathe.

Gaining Reach

There are several ways to increase your reach.

One way is to turn away from a hold and reach backwards for it. This is similar to reaching for something far under a bed.

Another method is to stand straight. Keep your hips close to the wall with your weight over your feet, as opposed to leaning against the rock.

Your last choice is bumping. This is where you gain momentum off one hold in order to reach a better one.

HOLDS AND GRIPS

Edges

An edge is a horizontal hold with a part you can grab onto. It's often flat, but sometimes has a lip you can pull on.

Crimp Grip

Crimping is grabbing the edge with your fingertips flat and your fingers arched above the tips. Crimping too hard can cause tendon damage.

Full Crimp

To do the full crimp, place the pads of your fingertips on an edge and curl your fingers so that the second joint is sharply flexed. Press your thumb on top of your index finger's fingernail to secure the grip.

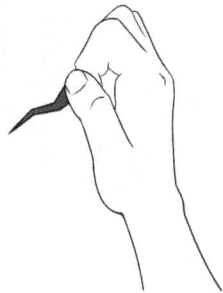

Half Crimp

If you let your thumb press against the side of your index finger, you are using the half crimp.

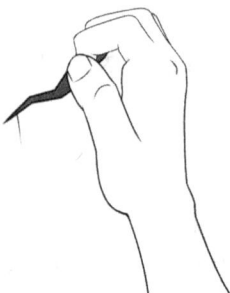

The half crimp is weaker, but less damaging to your fingers. If you have the option, use the half crimp.

Slopers

Slopers are rounded handholds without an edge. They're easiest to grab if they are above you. Keep your arms straight for maximum leverage when gripping them.

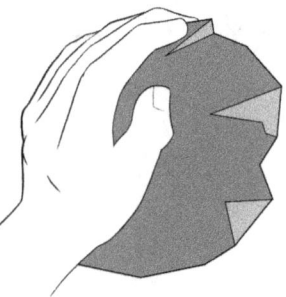

Open-hand Grip

To grab a sloper, use the open-hand grip.

Use the friction of your skin against the rock surface. Feel around with your fingers to find grip spots. Wrap your hand onto the hold, with your fingers close together, and then feel around with your thumb to see if there's a bump you can press against.

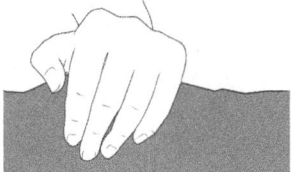

Pinches

Pinches are holds which can be gripped by pinching them with your fingers on one side and your thumb on the other.

If a pinch hold is small, use your thumb opposed to your index finger, with your middle finger stacked on top. With larger pinch holds, oppose your thumb with all your fingers.

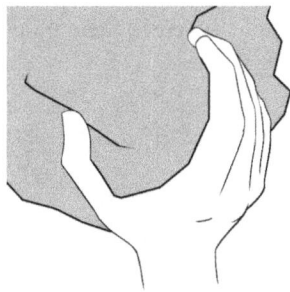

Side Pulls

Side pulls are holds that you pull sideways instead of straight down, due to their orientation. You can pull outward on the side pull while pushing a foot in the opposite direction to keep you in place.

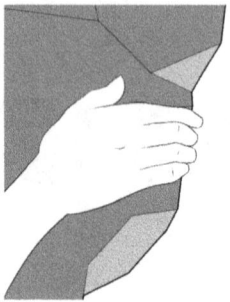

Pockets

Pockets are holes in the rock surface which you can place your finger(s) in.

Insert as many fingers as you can comfortably fit into a pocket. Use your strongest fingers first. Feel inside the pocket to find a surface you can pull against.

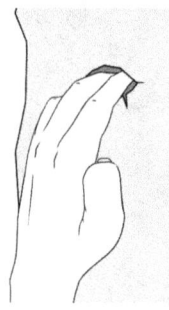

Gastons

A gaston is a hold oriented either vertically or diagonally, and is usually to your front.

Grab it with your fingers and palm facing into the rock and your thumb pointing downward. Bend your elbow at a sharp angle and point it away from your body. Crimp your fingers on the edge and pull outward.

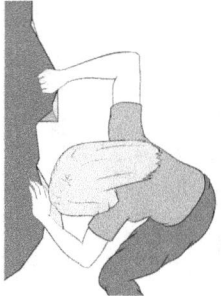

Undercling

An undercling is any hold that's gripped on its underside. It requires body tension and opposition.

Grip the rock with your palm facing up and your thumb pointing out. Pull out on the undercling and push your feet against the wall.

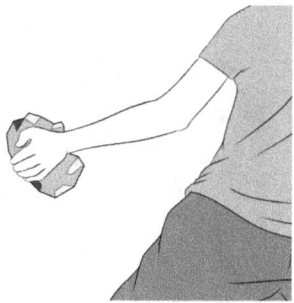

Palming

If no handhold exists, keep your hand in place by pushing into a dimple in the rock with the heel of your palm.

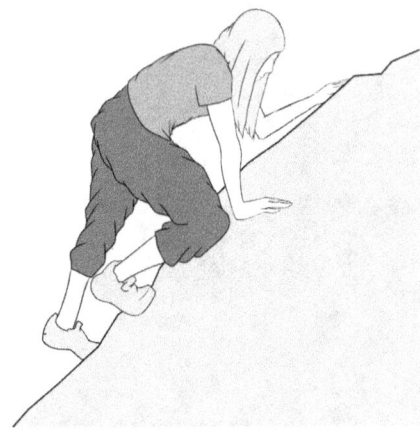

Matching Hands

Matching hands is when you place your hands next to each other on the same hold so you can change hands.

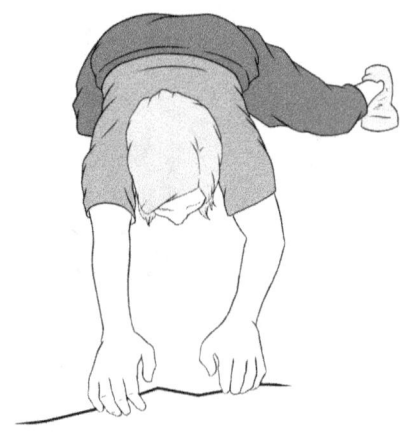

A similar technique can be done with your feet. Do so by slowly replacing one foot with the other and without jumping.

It can also be done with a hand and foot.

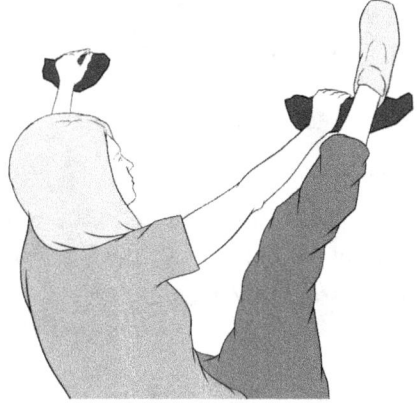

Plan ahead to minimize matching. For example, reach for an extra hold over so that your trailing hand can have its own hold.

FOOT TECHNIQUES

Smearing

To do this, push the flat of your foot hard on the wall, using friction to hold you up. If you want to go up, direct the force slightly downwards. Return to a foothold as soon as you can.

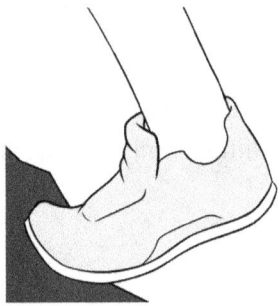

Back-stepping

To use this technique, step on a hold so that the outside of your hip faces into the rock, allowing for longer reach in the same direction as the foot that you stepped back with.

For an exaggerated back-step, drop one knee toward the ground with the other pointing up.

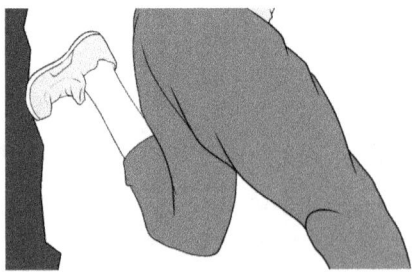

Flagging

Flagging is used to balance your body when reaching for a hold. Cross one foot behind the other to avoid swinging out from the rock.

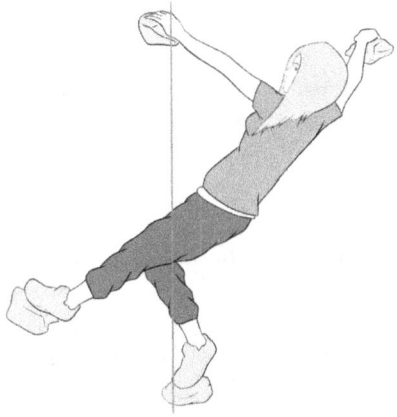

Stemming

Stemming is used to climb opposing walls, otherwise known as chimneys. Press a foot into one of the walls and your other foot against the other. Push out with opposing force to hold your weight up, and do the same with your hands.

Hold your weight with your arms/hands and shift both feet up. Once you have a good grip with your feet, hold your weight with your legs and move your hands up. Repeat this "shuffling" with your hands and feet to climb the chimney.

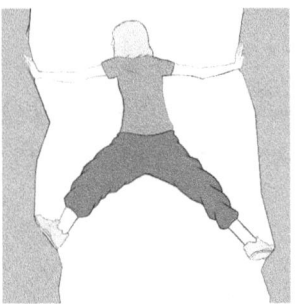

Hooking

Heel and toe hooks can aid in balance and provide leverage for movement.

There are a few ways to use a hook. For example, you can make one with your foot to climb onto a ledge.

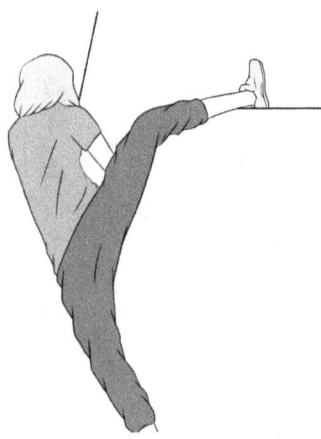

Hook under a rock to maintain your stability while you're negotiating an overhang.

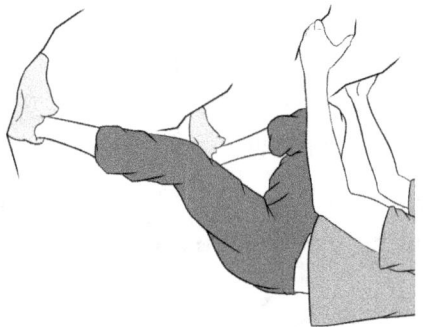

MANTLE

Use the mantle to climb up onto a ledge.

Get up close to the ledge. Pull yourself up, rock sideways, turn your hand around, and push yourself up until you can place a foot and stand up.

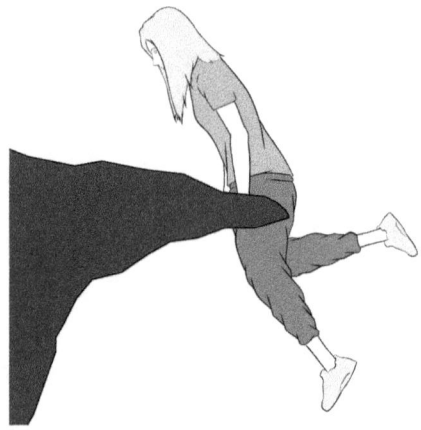

Exercises such as pulls-ups and muscle-ups will help build the strength needed to do mantles, which you can find in the Parkour section of this book.

Related Chapters:

- Pull-ups
- Muscle-ups

TYPES OF FACES

Slabs

A slab is any rock face than is angled at less than 90°.

To climb one, keep your weight centered on your feet. Stand upright on the rock and away from the slab surface.

Make small steps on small footholds rather than big steps on big holds. Plan the next three to five of your intended footholds ahead at a time. Aim for big holds and rest when you reach them.

As you climb, look for variations in the surface and smear on tiny holds.

Be precise with your toe placement. Feel the hold with a finger to find the best spot for your foot placement.

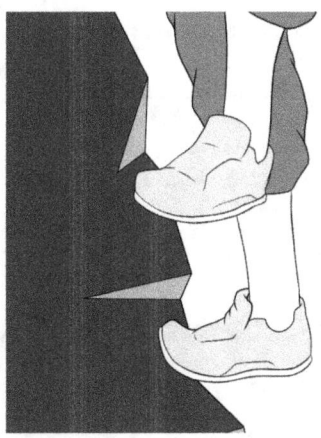

Vertical

Vertical faces are angled at 90°—that is, straight up (or close to it).

To climb one, keep your weight over your feet as much as possible. Use an upright body position, and use your hands and arms to pull if needed.

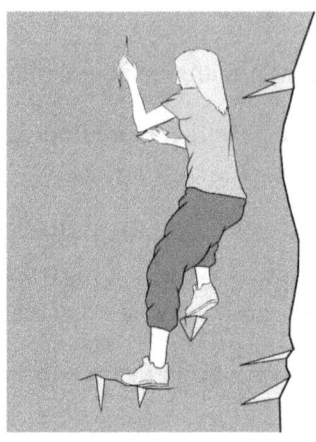

Overhangs

Overhangs are rock faces that are overhung or angled more than 90°.

When you're climbing them, heel and toe hooks are useful to take the weight off your arms.

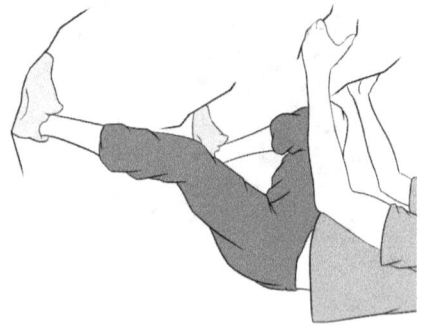

CRACK CLIMBING

Climb the natural cracks in the rock by jamming. Jamming is wedging your body parts into a crack. Doing so can cut your hands. Prevent this by taping your hands for protection.

Hand Jam

Wedge the side of your hand in the crack, with your thumb on top. Tuck your thumb into the palm of your hand.

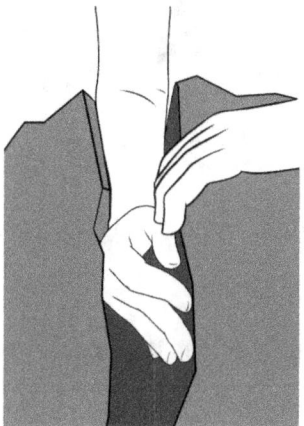

Expand your hand to exert opposing pressure against the walls of the crack. Hang your weight off your wedged hand.

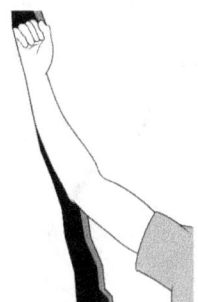

Foot Jam

Once your hands are jammed into the crack, lift a foot and push the front part of your shoe into the crack. Stand up on the jammed foot. Step the other foot up to calf level and jam it in the crack too.

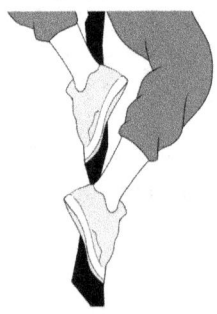

Shuffling

Move upward by shuffling your hands up the crack. There are three ways to do this:

- Move your top hand up first, then the lower one below it.
- Lift the bottom hand out of the crack and hand jam above your upper hand.
- Use the above two techniques together.

Do the same with your feet.

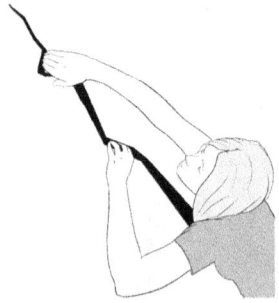

SWIMMING

This section has techniques and training methods for improving your ability in swimming:

- Quickly
- Long distances
- Underwater (speed and distance)

TREADING WATER

Treading water is the most energy-efficient way to stay in one spot. Learn to do so before doing any other water-based training. This is so that if you need to, you can tread water until you either create a plan for self-rescue or help arrives. When you're first learning, tread in shallow water and with a lifeguard present. Progress to deep water when you're confident.

While you're treading water, your body is vertical in the water and your head is above the surface. Your arms and legs work to keep you afloat. Torso movement is minimal.

There are a few ways to tread water. The following method is a little harder to get the hang of, but it's the most energy efficient. It combines vertical sculling with your arms and the eggbeater kick.

SCULLING

To scull, move your arms back and forth in the water, not up and down. Turn your palms in the direction that your arms are moving. Angle your thumbs up a little on the way in, and your pinky fingers up a little on the way out. Keep your back straight. Don't lean forward or backward.

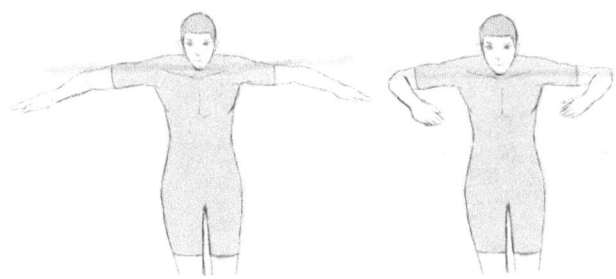

Vary the width of your stroke. Sometimes your hands should remain far apart, and sometimes they should almost come together.

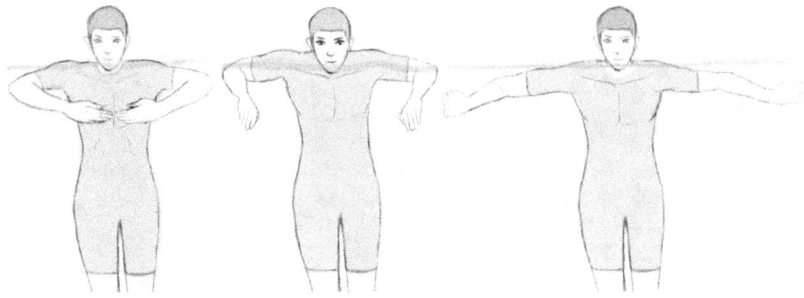

You can start by practicing this in shallow water. Find a depth where you can keep your head above water while you kneel. Begin the sculling action with your hands. Do it forcefully enough to raise your knees off the bottom.

When you're ready, move into deeper water. Place your feet directly underneath you, toes pointing straight down.

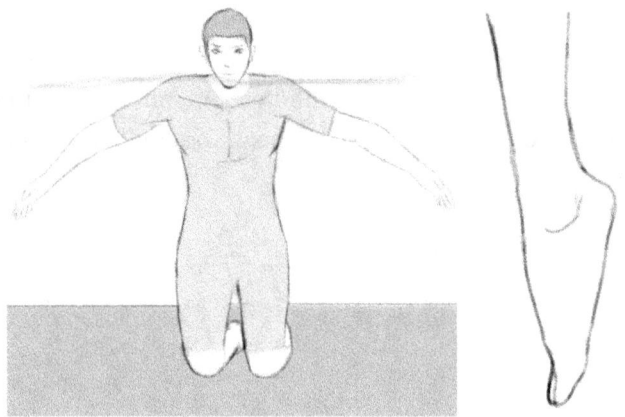

EGGBEATER KICK (ROTARY KICK)

The egg-beater kick can be tricky to learn, but it's worth going through the trouble. In comparison to the alternatives (such as the flutter kick), it's the most energy efficient.

Move your legs like an eggbeater, rotating each one in a different direction. It's like a breaststroke kick done one leg at a time. When one leg kicks out, the other should be coming in.

To begin learning the egg-beater kick, sit on the edge of a chair on dry land. Sit up straight and move only your right leg in a counter-clockwise circle. Next, move only your left leg in a clockwise circle. When you're ready, join these two leg movements together. As your right leg goes out, your left leg should come in, and vice versa.

Once you have the coordination, practice the egg-beater kick in the water. Lift your toes as you press down, so that your flat foot pushes down on the water, helping to propel you up. Point your toes as you bring your foot up, so that you have less resistance. Do not extend your legs completely. If they straighten out, you'll lose your upwards propulsion.

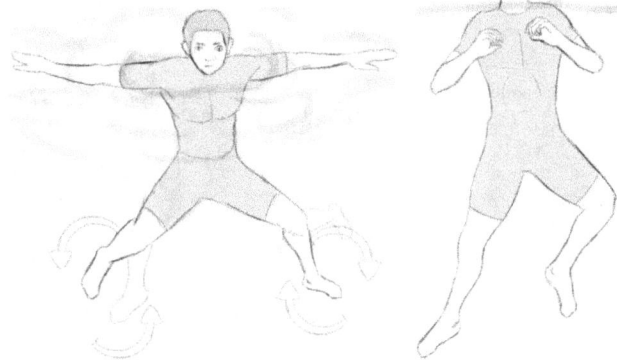

TREADING WATER

Once you're proficient at sculling and the eggbeater kick you can stay afloat by doing ONLY one or the other. You can perform tasks with your hands while staying afloat in one spot, and/or you can stay afloat in case of a leg injury.

By putting the two actions together, you'll conserve energy in both your arms and legs. This is ideal in a survival situation when you need to stay in one spot for long periods of time.

When treading water, stay calm and slow down your breathing. This will maximize your energy conservation.

Related Chapters:

- Sculling
- Eggbeater Kick (Rotary Kick)

SWIMMING QUICKLY

You will need to swim fast in emergency situations such as rescue or escape. Race swimming techniques are a base for this that you can then adapt for use in emergency situations.

There are three basic elements to consider when your goal is to swim quickly.

1. Entry and/or initial propulsion
2. Underwater swim
3. Surface swimming

Your initial propulsion is usually achieved by a dive entry or by pushing off something. Once you have your initial propulsion, you want to swim as fast and for as long as you can underwater. Use the fly-kick (either dolphin or fish tale). Swimming underwater is faster than surface swimming due to there being less resistance. When speed is your goal, swim underwater for as long as possible.

Once you need to surface for air, use freestyle (a.k.a. over-arm, front-crawl), since it's the fastest surface-swimming stroke.

It's assumed that you already know the basics of the three elements above. Now, we'll concentrate on improving the two factors needed to maximize speed for each element:

- Decreasing drag.
- Improving propulsion.

ENTRY AND INITIAL PROPULSION

You can use different entry and/or initial propulsion techniques depending on the situation. These techniques include:

- The push-off and streamlined position.
- The shallow dive.
- The dolphin dive.
- The deep-water floating start.
- The flip turn and push-off.

When speed is your primary goal, all these actions will lead into the underwater fly-kick.

Note: When you need to enter unknown waters, use the safe entry techniques described in part 2 of this manual. Opting for a safer entry technique may slow you down, but you won't be very fast at swimming if you get injured. Safety first, always.

Push-off and Streamlined Position

For the greatest speed when you're pushing off the edge, drop one to three feet below the water. When you're doing a flip turn, this will be automatic.

The best position for your legs/feet is shoulder width apart and with a bend in your knees. Push hard off the edge with strong legs and a tight core.

When you push off, your body must be as streamlined as possible. Become a straight arrow, stretching your body from your toes to your fingertips.

Place the palm of one hand on the back of the other. Wrap your upper hand's pinky and thumb around your lower hand, and then raise both hands over your head. Point your fingers in the direction you are going. Straighten your arms. Tuck them behind your head and squeeze your shoulder blades together. Another method is to squeeze your ears between your biceps.

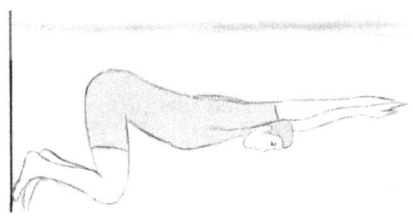

Keep your head down (swimming downhill), with the top of it pointing in the direction you want to go. Point your feet and turn your toes in towards each other a little (pigeon-toed). Keep your chin tucked and use a smooth exhale in whatever way is most comfortable for you.

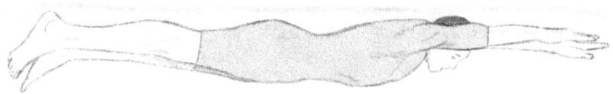

Maintain this streamline position as you push off the wall. Start the underwater fly-kick to maintain momentum underwater before surfacing into freestyle.

Note: Being on your side (as opposed to facing down) creates less resistance and may allow you to gain some speed. You should experiment with this.

Shallow Dive

Diving will give you the most propulsion, but is also the most dangerous entry method. **If you're unsure of the water depth and/or what lies below the surface, DO NOT DIVE!**

In an emergency, you may be pretty sure it's safe to dive, but not have the time for a thorough assessment. In this case, use the shallow dive. A shallow dive is one in which you arc into the water hands first while you adopt the streamlined position.

When you're starting to perfect your dive, do so from a stationary position. Place your lead (strongest) leg on the edge of the water (poolside, for example), with your toes a little over the edge. Your rear foot should be flat on the ground. Balance your weight evenly on both feet. Place your arms above your head in the streamlined position, with your chin tucked to your chest.

Push off with your lead foot so you get some distance. Arc over as you push and adopt the streamlined position as you enter the water.

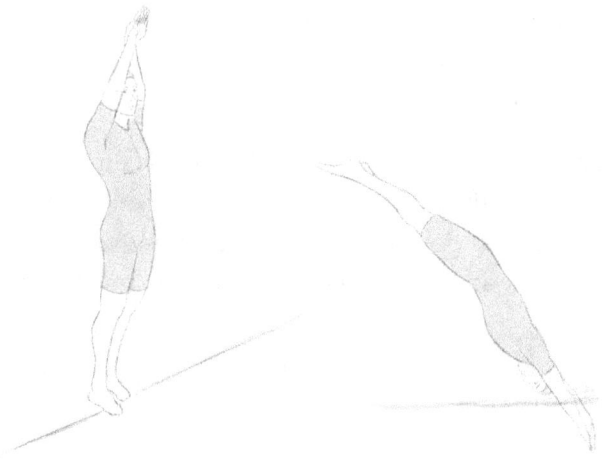

Once you are in the water, hold your head up and arch your back. This will steer your body up away from the bottom.

The more you arch, the more speed you will lose. You have to compromise depending on the water depth. Remember that you will be faster streamlining a couple of feet below the surface.

Note: Do not look/arch up before you are in the water. You will lose speed and may get injured.

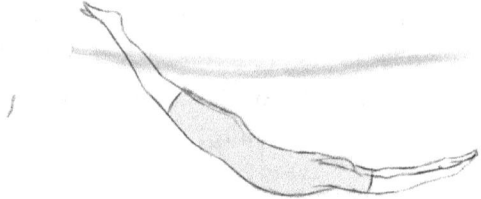

When you're ready, try diving from a walking and then a running start. In these cases, your arms will start by your sides. Once you leap off the edge, adopt the correct position so you can enter the water using the same basic form.

Dolphin Dive

Dolphin dives are useful when running into the water from a beach. They'll allow you to overcome waist/chest deep water as fast as possible. To preserve your forward momentum, run until the water is knee or waist high, and then use a dolphin dive.

As you run in, look out for obstacles in the terrain, such as rocks or holes. Once you hit the water, lift your feet completely out of the water for as long as possible. This will decrease your drag time. Put your hands in the streamlined position and leap/arc over into a dive.

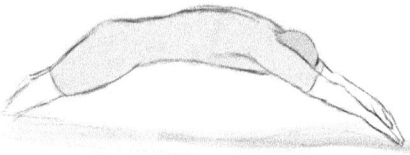

Don't dive too hard, or you might injure yourself, but dive deep enough to reach the sand on the bottom. Grab hold of the sand and lock your feet one in front of the other. Push forward off the ground into your next dolphin dive as fast as you can. Continue to dolphin dive in rapid succession until it's too deep to continue (about neck deep).

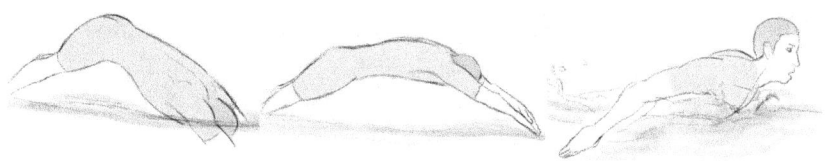

Do not look up while dolphin diving. As with the shallow dive, this is important for safety and speed.

If a wave is approaching, dolphin dive under it, grab the sand and stay under until the wave passes over you.

Once it's too deep to dolphin dive, transition into the underwater flykick.

You can also use the dolphin dive to come back into shore. Swim until it's shallow enough to dolphin dive, then continue to dolphin dive until you can run out.

Floating Start

Use a floating start from a floating/treading position when you have nothing to push off. The key for this is to use an explosive initial kick (such as a side scissor kick) and then go straight into freestyle. If you know that you will need a floating start, get as close to the freestyle position as possible.

Adopt a horizontal position. Place your dominant hand in front, ready to pull back into your first stroke. Have your other arm in a half-stroke position. Your heels should be close to the surface of the water. Tread water in this position.

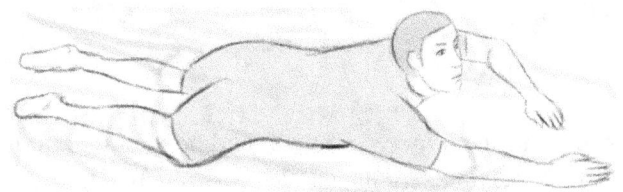

When it's time to swim, kick hard as you pull with your first stroke and transition into normal freestyle.

Flip Turns

Flip turns are often identified with swimming races in a pool. Having to turn in the water in an emergency is not likely, but it is possible. Knowing how to flip turn will make it much faster for you to do this.

First, learn the flip turn without having to push off the wall. In an emergency, this is most likely the style you will use.

The main flip part of the flip turn is actually only a half-flip. Start by swimming on your stomach (freestyle, for example). As your arm enters the water for the turn, start a half-flip by tucking your chin and doing a small dolphin kick. At the same time, move your hands to your sides. Breathe out through your nose to prevent any water getting up it.

Continue the half-flip by tucking your knees towards your eyes and your feet to your bum. At the same time, push down with the palms of your hands to get your feet over your head. Keep your elbows close to your body while doing this.

As you complete the half-flip, bring your arms into the streamlined position. You are now pointing in your new travel direction.

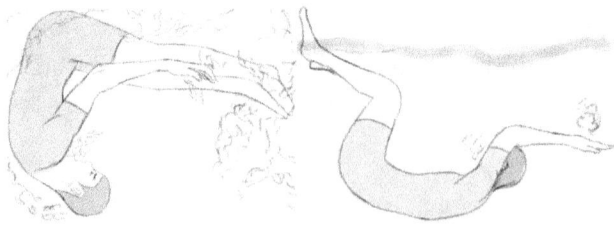

Roll onto your stomach by twisting your hands a little and looking in the direction you want to rotate. Don't turn your head; just move your eyes.

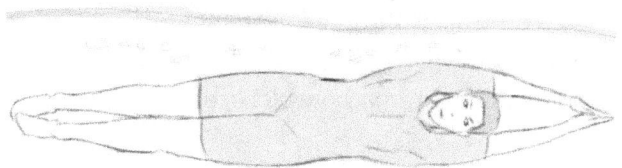

Use an explosive kick and arm pull to set you off in your new direction like you would in a floating start.

Note: Don't try to look where you are going during the flip. It will slow you down and mess up your coordination. Look at your knees instead.

To turn and push off a wall (such as in a pool swimming race) speed up (kick harder) when you are about five meters away from the wall. Ensure you have enough air to make the turn, but don't take a breath before it, as you'll slow down.

Once you are a bit more than an arm's length away from the wall, do the turn as normal. Push off the wall as described before (Push-off/Streamlined Position). The difference is that you'll be face up when you do the push-off, with your toes pointing up.

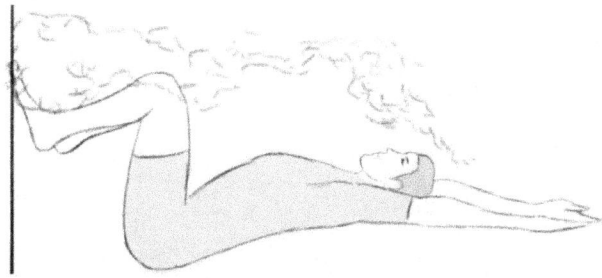

Once you push off, start to turn onto your stomach and then do underwater fly-kicks. You may wish to start to fly-kick before (whilst on your back), and/or during your turn. Experiment to discover what you prefer/works best for you. Continue to fly-kick until you need to start surface swimming.

Once you can do the basic turn and push off, work on perfecting your distance in relation to the wall. Land on your feet, with your knees bent close to 90° and your hips bent close to 110°.

Related Chapters:

- Underwater Fly-Kick
- Freestyle
- Safety

UNDERWATER FLY-KICK

When you know how to do it, swimming underwater is faster than swimming on the surface. When you want to go fast, swim underwater for as long as you can.

The fastest way to swim underwater is using the underwater fly-kick. There are two main ways to do the underwater fly-kick: the dolphin kick and the fish kick. If you're good at it, the fish kick is faster than the dolphin kick, but in the Survival Fitness Plan (SFP), we focus on the dolphin kick because it is:

- Easier to master.
- Easier to control, especially in open water.
- Used in other strokes outlined in this manual.

Once you have the standard dolphin kick mastered, you may wish to progress to the fish kick. After your initial propulsion (e.g., dive or push-off), maintain your streamlined position. You want to maximize this glide phase before you start kicking.

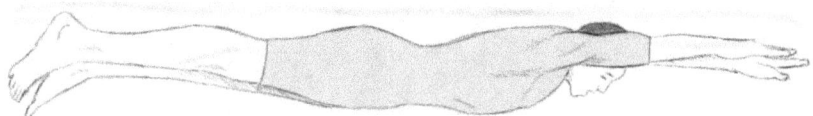

Just before you start to slow down, kick up and down with both feet/legs at the same time. Keep your upper body in the streamline position.

Bend your knees so that your kicks start and finish well in front of (or behind) your body, but do not kick from your knees. Use your core/hips to generate the power. To do this, suck in your stomach and squeeze your buttocks together.

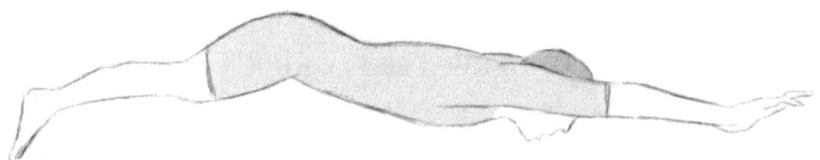

You must also snap your toes and ankle. It may help to think of your body as a whip. The power comes from your core (the handle), and your feet/toes are the tip of the whip, which snaps up and down. Kick fast and kick small. Ensure you also kick backward instead of only up and down. You want to push the water behind you. Your up and down kicks should be of equal force. Use the vertical kicking drill to develop your coordination and strength for this. The vertical kicking drill is in the Freestyle chapter.

When you start to surface, begin freestyle swimming.

Ankle Strength and Flexibility

Increasing your ankle strength and flexibility will improve your dolphin (and flutter) kick. Here are some exercises you can do:

Ankle rotations. Move your foot and ankle in a circle as large as possible without pain. Do 15–20 circles in each direction.

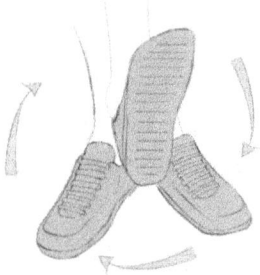

Ankle stretches. There are four levels of this exercise. Each increases in difficulty from the previous one. From a standing position, place the top of your toes on the ground a half step behind your other foot. Push down and forward into the ground. Sit on your heels, with your shins and the tops of your feet flat on the ground.

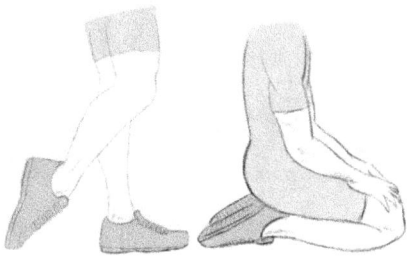

Lean back onto your hands to increase the stretch. Finally, put your hands up in the streamlined position and then lift your knees off the ground.

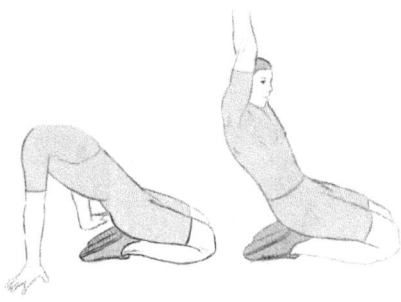

Ankle Inversion. From a standing position, roll one foot to the outside. Press the edge of your foot into the ground gently. Only do one foot at a time.

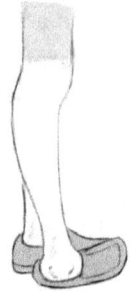

Related Chapters:

- Freestyle

FREESTYLE

This chapter assumes you already know the basic mechanics of swimming freestyle.

Freestyle (overarm) is the fastest way to surface-swim. By improving your technique, you will become faster and more energy efficient. There are a few different areas you can tweak. Practice in each individual area, and then put them all together when you're ready.

Balance

Being balanced in the water will make you more streamlined and so will increase your speed. Maintain a position that is as close to horizontal as possible.

Except when taking a breath, keep your head down and your neck relaxed. Imagine you have a blowhole in the back of your neck that you have to keep open. Looking down (as opposed to forwards) will also help.

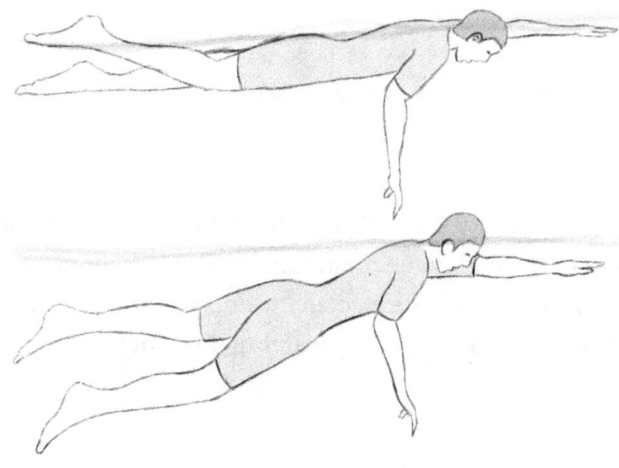

Breathing

Breathing while swimming (as opposed to holding your breath underwater) increases your stamina. Start blowing out as soon as you finish inhaling, and continue to do so until you take your next breath.

Experiment with breathing rhythms (take a breath every third or fifth stroke, for example) to see what works best for you. It may help to count your arm strokes (1, 2, 3, 4, breathe, for instance).

It is important to exhale completely before taking your next breath, so that you get rid of all the stale air. This increases your stamina and keeps you streamlined for longer. Every time you breathe, you break your streamline position.

Keep as close to your streamline position as possible while breathing. Do this by turning your head as opposed to lifting it out of the water. Your mouth only needs to be a little ways out of the water for you to inhale. Your eyeline should be no higher than the surface. If you're looking to the sky, you're turning your head way too much.

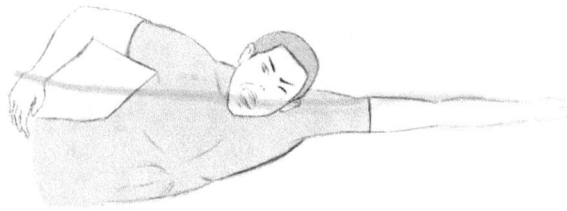

Breathing on alternate sides of your body (bilaterally) is a good habit. Always inhale through your mouth, but try to exhale most of the air through your nose. This is especially useful when you're turning/flipping, as it helps you avoid getting water up your nose.

Rolling

Roll from side to side with each arm stroke. This will engage your back muscles and improve propulsion. Engage your core as you do it.

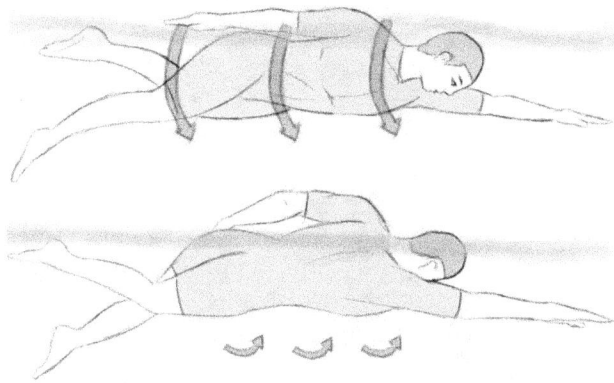

The following drill is good for getting used to floating on your sides.

Float flat on your back and do a light flutter kick for propulsion. Keep your body straight, with your arms at your sides. Apply downward pressure on the back of your head and on your shoulder blades, so that your hips and legs buoy up.

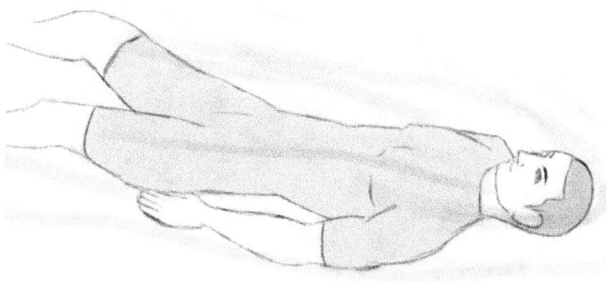

Once you feel balanced in this position, do the following:

- Roll onto your side so that your top arm and some of your top thigh clear the water.
- Do not move your while you roll on your side. Keep looking at the sky and roll your body as one.
- Continue to flutter kick.

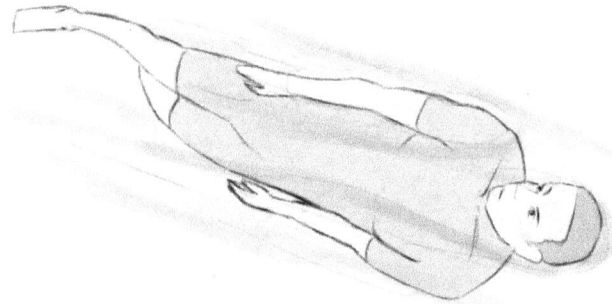

Roll as far as you're comfortable. A 45° body roll is good for most people.

Practice this on both sides of your body. Once you are comfortable with the above, advance by rolling to 90°, so that you face down.

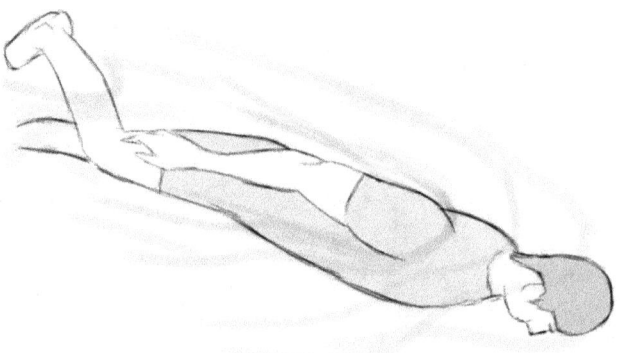

Keep flutter kicking, and keep balanced. Continue to roll in the same direction until you're in the 45° position, but on your opposite side. Remember to roll your whole body together. Don't lead with your head. When you're balanced, roll back the other way.

Arm Technique

The freestyle stroke is explained in four parts: the catch, pull, exit, and recovery. These four stages occur and repeat in the order listed.

There is a more advanced arm stroke known as the early vertical forearm position (EVF). It is harder to master, holds a greater risk of injury, and offers a minimal gain in speed. It's more for elite competitive swimmers. The following technique is like a non-extreme EVF.

THE CATCH is when your hand first enters the water.

Create a web with your hand by spreading your fingers apart a little, about 30% of the diameter of one finger. Maintain this spacing the whole time.

As you roll your body, stretch your arm out, with your palm faced down. Angle your fingertips downward a little and flex your wrist. Point your middle finger in the direction you'll travel. Place your hand in the water fingertips first. Ensure your arm/hand doesn't cross your centerline.

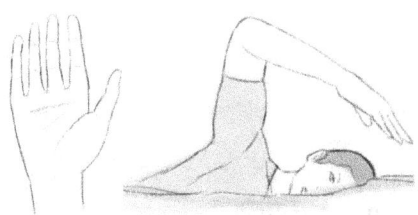

Once your hand is in the water, bend your elbow and press back on the water. Your forearm is in a near-vertical position. Don't push forward once your hand is in the water; it's better to go straight into the pull phase of the stroke. It may help to imagine your arm is moving over a big ball.

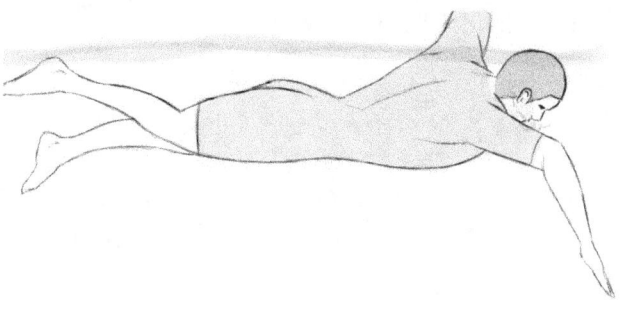

You can use finger paddles to help you perfect your catch. Wear them loosely. If you over-reach or have some other bad technique, the paddles will come off.

Another thing you can do is use a kickboard. Focus on making a good catch with only one arm. The kickboard will prevent you from reaching forward.

THE PULL is the movement of your arm in the water down the length of your body. After you make a good catch, your elbow will be in the "high" position. It will face the sky, while your palm faces to your rear. Keep this high elbow as you push the water behind you.

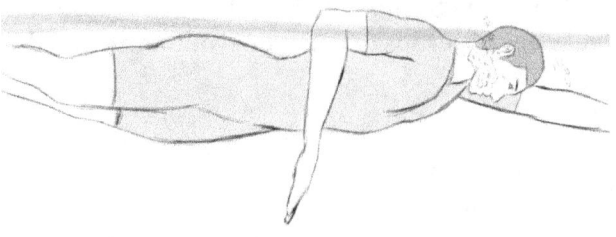

A good catch and pull is an easy, flowing feeling. You get great forward propulsion using your pecs and lats.

THE EXIT phase of your stroke is when your arm/hand leaves the water just past your hip.

It's important not to be too eager to bring your arm out of the water. Push beyond your hip as if you're trying to reach your knee, using the same press-up motion you would when exiting a pool using the wall. Do this push for the whole range of your pull, and as your thumb touches your thigh, flick the water out.

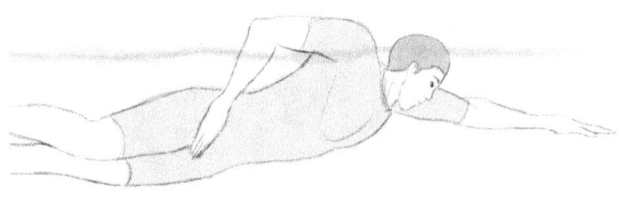

THE RECOVERY is the time when your arm is in the air. Your arm flicks out of the exit and then re-enters into the catch. It's best not to think about your recovery. Let it take its natural path. Your mental effort is better spent focusing on a great catch.

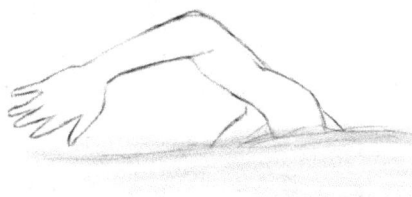

You can use stretch cords to practice all phases of your stroke on dry land. They're also useful for focusing on problem areas.

Efficient Kicking

A good kick is a compact one. It shouldn't be too low or break the water's surface. Don't disturb your natural alignment. Move your feet/legs independently of each other. Push one down as you pull the other up. Putting energy into both the up and down strokes is important.

Use short, quick kicks with your whole leg, starting at the hip. Keep your legs long and straight, but not rigid. Have a slight, natural bend in your knees. Point your toes behind you, but keep your ankles relaxed. Only the bottoms of your feet should meet the water's surface. Find a rhythm that's comfortable and stick with it. Around 15 kicks every 10 seconds is good.

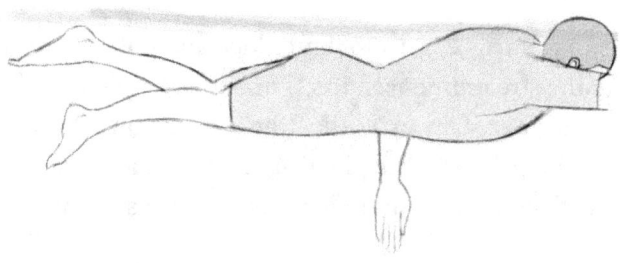

This vertical kicking drill will help to improve your flutter kick. It's also good for your dolphin kick. Do this drill in deep water, but make sure you are near something you can hold onto when you get tired.

Position yourself vertically in the water and do nothing but flutter kick to keep your mouth and nose above the surface. You will be kicking hard. Concentrate on the correct kicking technique, as described above. Begin with your arms underwater, and use a small sculling motion.

As you improve, try keeping your arms and hands tight against your body.

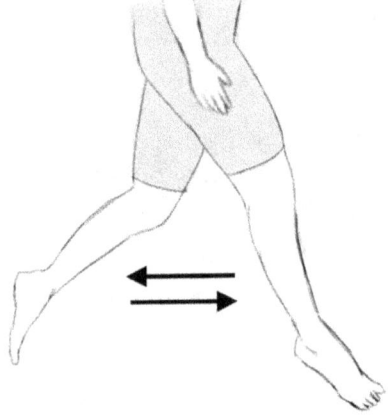

Advance further by raising your fingertips out of the water. Raise your arms higher and higher as you gain strength.

Transitioning from the Fly Kick to Freestyle

As you begin to surface, start to flutter kick and pull one of your arms down from the streamline position. Time the completion of your pull phase so that your arm exits the water as if you had been doing freestyle all along. This takes practice. Complete a few strokes before taking a breath, and then continue into freestyle as normal.

Additional Tips for Improvement

You can adapt most of these tips to all areas of swimming, and life in general.

- **Train regularly,** at least twice a week.
- **Compete against your times.** Notice what causes you to swim faster, and use what works best for you.
- **Identify and work on your weak points.**
- **Visualize someone chasing you.** Imagine you are being chased, then work on calming your mind and body and concentrate on swimming as fast as you can.
- **Get a professional swim coach.** Those of you who are having difficulties or want to get to the next level may benefit from guidance.

SWIMMING LONG DISTANCES

There are two strokes to learn for long-distance swimming: the survival backstroke and the combat sidestroke.

The survival backstroke, a.k.a. the elementary backstroke, is an easy to learn and is very energy efficient. It is for long-distance and/or survival situations, such as when waiting for rescue.

The combat side stroke (CSS) is an ultra-efficient variation of the sidestroke. It was developed by the Navy SEALS and is perfect for escape, evasion, and survival.

- It is efficient (fast yet energy conserving).
- You can do it with gear (like a backpack).
- Your body profile is lower (you'll be harder to see).
- It's excellent for swimming through the surf in open water.
- You can observe your surroundings as you swim, unlike with the survival backstroke.

SURVIVAL BACKSTROKE

This chapter assumes you know the basic mechanics of the survival backstroke.

The survival backstroke involves floating on your back as you propel yourself through the water. You use a simultaneous frog/breaststroke kick and a sculling motion with your hands. Your arms and legs move and come together at the same time.

The main goal of the survival backstroke is to conserve energy and reduce heat loss. To maximize energy conservation, do the survival backstroke very slowly. Take short strokes and glide for as long as possible. Only take the next stroke when you feel your legs dropping or you lose forward momentum.

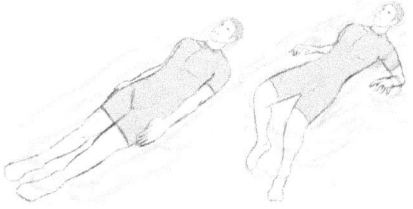

Taking short strokes minimizes heat loss from under your armpits and between your legs. Your arms should not extend beyond your shoulders. At the end of each stroke, bring your arms and legs together. Hold them close, but comfortably, against your body.

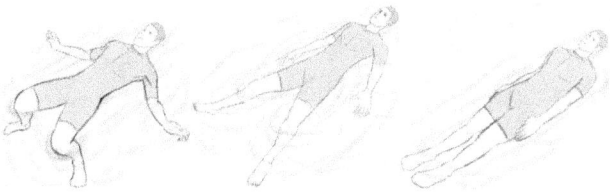

Use the survival backstroke is if an underwater explosion is likely. You will want to go faster so you can escape the blast, so make your strokes larger. Take your next stroke sooner than normal, but not too soon. Make the most out of your streamlined glide position while achieving the most speed.

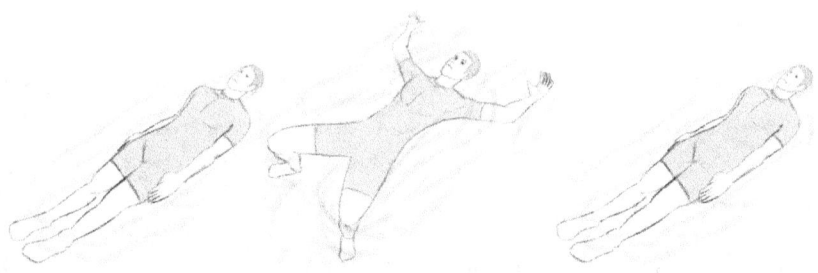

Related Chapters:

- Sculling

COMBAT SIDESTROKE

The combat sidestroke (CSS) is a mix of freestyle, breaststroke, and sidestroke. There are four basic stages to the CSS: the streamline position, two catch and pull movements, and the recovery. The recovery involves a scissor kick paired with a breaststroke-like arm movement.

Note: A lot of the terminology used in this chapter is explained in the Freestyle chapter.

Streamline Position

Get some initial propulsion. Adopt the streamline position, as explained in the Entry and Initial Propulsion chapter.

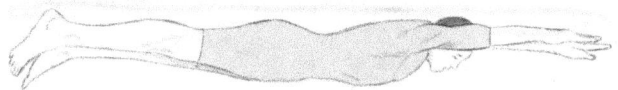

First Catch and Pull

Do your first catch by pressing the palm of your top hand down. If you are rolling to your right, then your right hand should be on top. Bend your arm at the elbow.

Make sure to keep your arm aligned at a downward angle. Your shoulder should be at the top, your elbow below that, then your wrist, and finally your fingers at the bottom. Doing this will maximize your first pull.

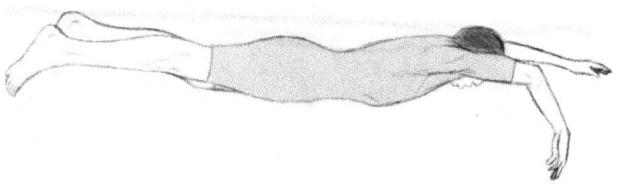

Continue the catch as you rotate onto your side. Your forearm should be positioned vertically, with your elbow above your wrist. Stay on your side until your recovery stage.

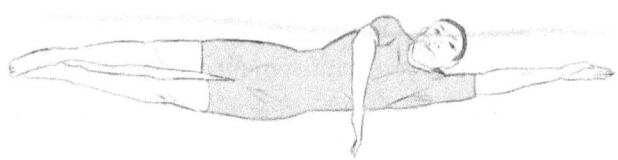

Flow into the pull by continuing the movement of your top arm until your hand is in line with your upper thigh. Your hand should follow your midline. Be careful not to raise your elbow too high.

At this stage, your arm should be almost fully extended. Do not let your hand come out of the water. Now is a good time to take a breath. When you exhale, do so slowly and steadily.

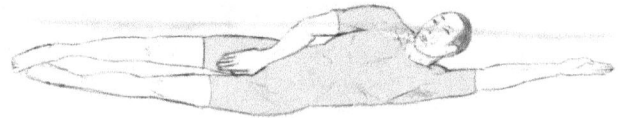

Second Catch and Pull

Start your second catch and pull with your other arm by sweeping it down. Your palm should face down and stay fixed in that position. As you sweep down, it will create resistance against the water, propelling you forward.

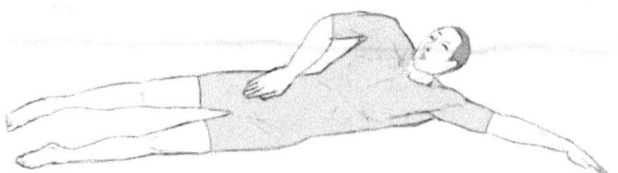

When your arm is vertical, your palm will be facing to your rear. Continue the arc of your bottom arm until your hand is on your thigh.

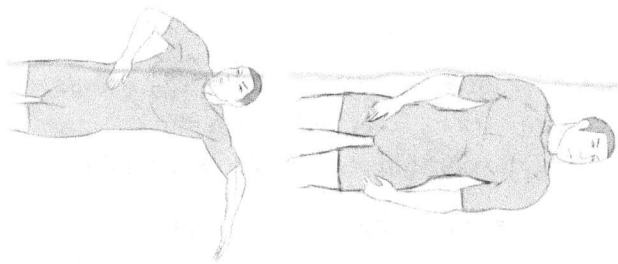

The catch, pull, and recovery of your lower arm is almost identical to a breaststroke motion.

Note: As you do the second pull you can either leave your head up breathing or look back down. If you tend to sink, you're better off looking back down.

Recovery

Start the recovery with a simultaneous scissor kick and arm movement.

Bring both your arms up through the centerline of your body, then back into the streamline position, like breaststroke. Keep your arms and hands underwater and as close to your body as possible. Move your arms forward past your face as you do the scissor kick. Finish in the streamline position.

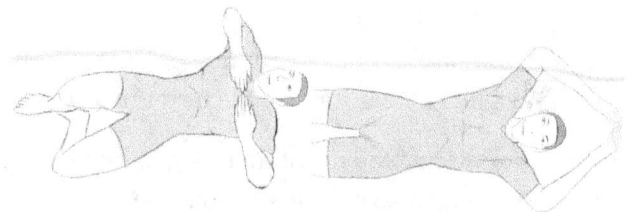

Scissor Kick

Do the scissor kick as you bring your arms forward. This helps with propulsion and corkscrews your body back into the streamline position.

Move your top leg forward and your bottom leg backward at the same time. Bring them back together in the streamline position. Keep your toes flexed towards your shin until you adopt that position.

Draw your top knee up so there is a 90° angle at your hip and knee. At the same time, bend your bottom leg back at the knee. Extend the lower part of your top leg in front of your torso as you kick your bottom leg back.

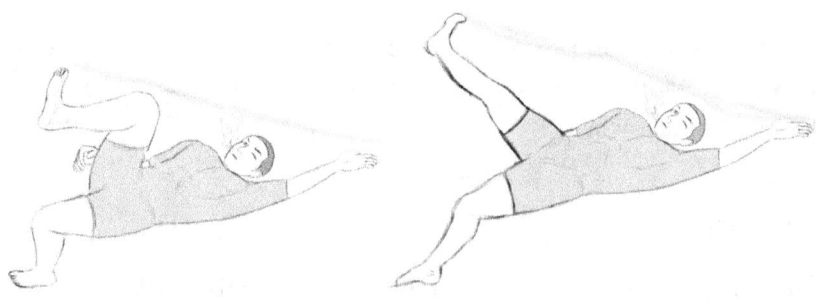

Point your toes once you have extended your legs, then draw them into the streamline position.

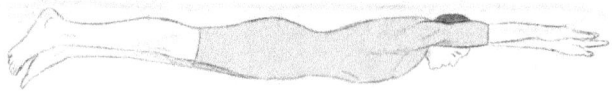

Slowly exhale as you glide in the streamline position. Be sure to get the most out of the glide before starting the next arm cycle.

If speed is more important, you can flutter kick before initiating your first pull again. You could also use the sprinter's CSS.

Sprinter's CSS

Use the sprinter's CSS when you need to go faster. The tradeoff is that you'll use more energy, since you'll have a greater stroke count over the same distance.

To do the sprinter's CSS, do a half-stroke on your second pull. Everything else will stay the same. From the start of the second pull, bring your arm down as normal, until it's almost at a right angle to your body. Instead of pulling it all the way to your thigh, scoop it up into your armpit.

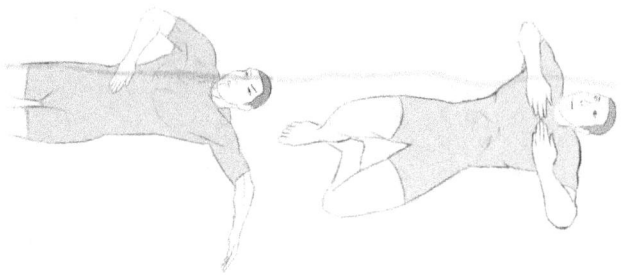

From here, push it forward into a full extension as normal.

Guide Stroke

Use the guide stroke to check your direction when using the CSS to swim a long distance. It uses a breaststroke-type movement for your arms and the dolphin kick for your legs.

Start in the streamline position. Push your palms out against the water to a position a little wider than your shoulders.

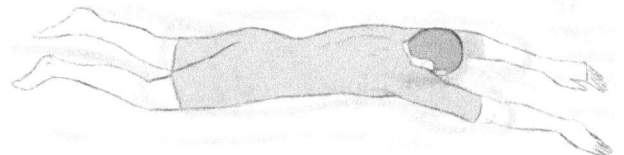

Press your palms against the water as you rotate your hands and lower arms into a vertical position. Your fingertips should point down, and your palms should be angled toward your chest.

Pull your palms towards your chest. This creates forward propulsion and allows you to raise your head above the surface. Now you can breathe and look around, but try not to lift your head too far out of the water, as this will cause your hips and legs to sink, and decrease your momentum.

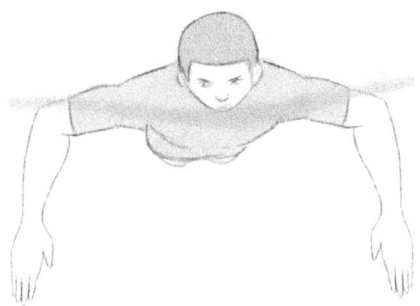

Move your arms back to the streamline position as you would with breaststroke. Keep them close to your body along your centerline.

As you recover your arms, use the downward motion of the dolphin kick. This helps with propulsion back into the streamline position. From here, you can continue into CSS or another guide stroke.

Note: For more instruction on the dolphin kick, see the underwater fly-kick chapter.

If you get disoriented, tread water until you figure out which direction you need to swim in.

Related Chapters:

- Entry and Initial Propulsion
- Underwater Fly-Kick
- Freestyle

SWIMMING LONG DISTANCES UNDERWATER

There are two major factors when it comes to swimming long distances underwater:

1. Efficient stroke.
2. Lung capacity (how long you can hold your breath).

This section offers a five stage-training plan. Use it to increase your ability to swim long distances underwater.

Important note: Depriving yourself of oxygen is dangerous. Safe training is paramount!

SAFETY

Here are some safety pointers to keep in mind when you're practicing to swim long distances underwater:

- Train with a partner, and not at the same time. Your friend must watch you so he can help if something goes wrong. If you must train alone, then at least make sure there is a lifeguard present.
- Stay in shallow water, especially to begin with.
- Never push yourself to beat your last time or distance. Only hold your breath for as long as is comfortable. Trying to beat your record will have an adverse effect anyway. You're much better off staying relaxed and seeing where you pop up.
- If you begin to panic at any moment, relax and surface.
- Listen to your body. If you get light-headed, your vision begins to fade, or you get any other abnormal sensation, surface immediately.
- Work on your lung capacity on dry land, and concentrate more on making efficient strokes when you're in the water.

STAGE ONE: DRY-LAND BREATH-HOLDING

Practice holding your breath for longer periods of time while you're on dry land.

In the Survival Fitness Plan, we use minimal preparation for breath-holding. This is so you know how far you can get in emergency situations. Breathe in, breathe out, breathe in, then go.

Take these breaths slowly, from deep within your diaphragm. This is to rid your lungs of low-quality air (CO_2).

You know you're using correct breathing if your belly, not your shoulders, is moving up and down. When your chest and shoulders move, it means you're breathing with only the top part of your lungs. This deeper breathing is also useful for recovery after a workout.

While doing the following, relax your muscles and remain as still and as calm as possible. Don't do any clock-watching, as it will make you anxious. The more relaxed and still you are, the less oxygen your body will consume.

Follow these detailed instructions for the inhale, exhale, inhale, sequence:

- Breathe in for a count of 5 seconds, hold for 1 second, then breathe out for a count of 10 seconds.
- When exhaling, push out every last drop of air, and push your tongue up against your teeth. This forms a valve which helps to control the release of air. Your breath should make a hissing sound as you exhale.
- Inhale slowly, to about 80–85% capacity. Start at the bottom, near your diaphragm, then up into your sternum, and finally into your chest.
- Hold your breath for as long as you can, and when you first

start to feel the need to breathe, swallow a little spit. This helps to relax your breathing reflex.
- When you need to breathe out, let out little puffs of air at a time.
- When you're finished, push out as much air as possible to get rid of any extra carbon dioxide.

Don't try this sequence again until you get your body back to normal oxygen levels. Breathe steadily for at least five minutes, and don't do it more than three times in a single session. Only do one session a day.

After a few practice sessions, try adding in slow movements, such as walking. This will prepare your body to dive and swim with less air.

STAGE TWO: STATIC UNDERWATER BREATH-HOLDING

Stage two is the same as stage one, but underwater. The point of this stage is to get you comfortable holding your breath underwater.

Inhale, exhale fully, inhale to 80% capacity, then hold and submerge. Keep your mouth and nose closed while underwater. Use your fingers to hold your nose shut if you need to.

Stay relaxed, and resurface once you're near your limit. Blow out any extra air as you rise, so that you can take a fresh breath immediately.

STAGE THREE: STATIC APNEA TRAINING

In this stage, you will use static apnea training. This conditions your lungs and body to withstand the effects of prolonged breath-holding. This stage is ongoing. You can move on to stage 4 while doing it.

Important note: This is a dry land activity. DO NOT try it underwater!

There are two separate programs for static apnea training. One increases your CO_2 tolerance. The other increases the amount of oxygen your lungs can store.

Each program has its own training table. The recovery stage is when you can breathe normally for the allotted time. During the breath-hold stage, hold your breath for the allotted time. Only start O_2 tolerance training once you can hold your breath for at least 90 seconds. You can do both CO_2 and O_2 sessions on the same day, but do not do them immediately after one another. Do one in the morning and one at night. Do not do more than one of each per day.

CO2 Tolerance

CO_2 tolerance training consists of a series of alternating breath-holds and rest periods. Your breathing time gets shorter, while the time you hold your breath holding stays the same. Start off with a breath-holding period that you're comfortable with. Try 50-70% of the maximum time you can hold it. Add 5 or 10 seconds each day.

The table below outlines one training session in which you recover and hold your breath eight times. Use the same breath hold time for each one. In your next training session (the following day), increase the time you hold your breath by 5 or 10 seconds.

#	Recovery	Breath Hold
1	2m 30s	50-70%
2	2m 15s	50-70%
3	2m	50-70%
4	1m 45s	50-70%
5	1m 30s	50-70%
6	1m 15s	50-70%
7	1m	50-70%
8	45s	50-70%

O2 Tolerance

In O2 tolerance training, your recovery period stays the same. Instead, you increase your breath holding.

Only start O2 tolerance training once you can hold your breath for at least 90 seconds.

This table shows one training session.

#	Recovery	Breath Hold
1	2m	50%
2	2m	55%
3	2m	60%
4	2m	65%
5	2m	70%
6	2m	75%
7	2m	80%
8	2m	85%

Additional Ways to Increase Your Breath-Holding Ability

There are some other things you can do to increase your breath-holding ability:

- Exercise often.
- Lose weight if you are overweight.
- Learn to play a wind or brass instrument.
- Take up singing.
- Don't do drugs, and especially avoid smoking!

Body Response Information

This is for informational purposes. DO NOT practice/experiment with it.

When you hold your breath for an extended period, your body goes through three response stages:

1. **Convulsions.** When you first get an urge to take a breath and you don't, you will have convulsions in your diaphragm. You can learn to fight through this, and if you do, you will gain a couple of minutes before you need to breathe.
2. **Spleen release.** If you fight through the convulsions your spleen responds by releasing oxygen-rich blood. Your body will calm down and you'll get a surge of energy. Use this energy to get somewhere that you can breathe!
3. **Blackout.** If you do not find fresh oxygen, you will black out. If you're underwater at the time, you'll drown.

STAGE FOUR: EFFICIENT STROKE

This teaches the technique for an efficient underwater stroke. The only aim is to learn the stroke. Don't try to break any underwater distance records. This stroke uses a combination of a modified breaststroke (for the arms) and the dolphin kick. Do it as one fluid motion. Start off in a streamlined glide and stay in it for as long as possible.

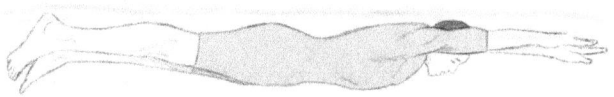

When you are almost to a complete stop, turn your palms out and separate your hands. Do the out-sweep of the breaststroke. Use webbed fingers, as described in the Freestyle chapter (under the heading Catch). Allow your legs to float up—the higher the better. Keep your head down.

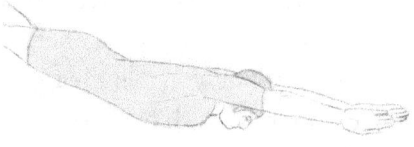

As you do the breaststroke arm movement, arch your body, extending your back and shoulders. You aim is to make your body like a spring that you'll snap down to propel you forward. Bring your arms and forearms into a vertical position, elbows facing up. Snap your arms and legs down together.

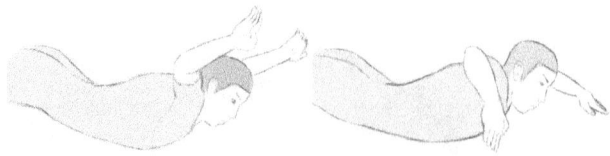

Do a dolphin kick and go into a double-armed pull stroke by pushing against the water down along your body. Remember your webbed fingers.

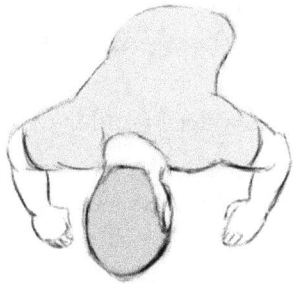

Keep your arms vertical for as long as you can and end in a streamline position with your arms by your sides. Glide in this position for as long as you can.

Do a standard breaststroke frog kick. At the same time, bring your hands back into the streamline glide you started in, with your arms/hands in front of you.

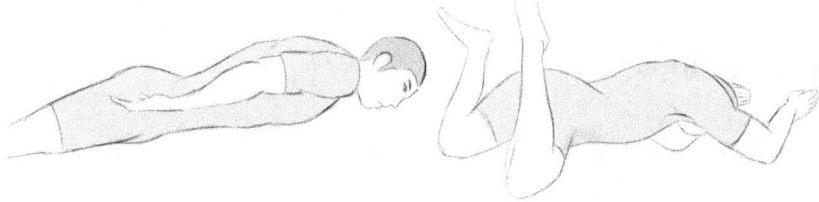

Repeat this sequence. When you start to run out of breath, go into your preferred surface stroke. CSS or freestyle is best.

Related Chapters:

- Freestyle

STAGE FIVE: 50M SWIM

Revisit the safety pointers from the start of this section.

Before attempting this final stage, you should be able to:

- Swim 25 meters underwater in under 30 seconds, using 5 strokes or less.
- Hold your breath for at least 90 seconds while walking on dry land.

The first part of stage five is building up your breath holding ability while moving on dry land. Hold your breath while doing SFP super-burpees for a minute. When you can do six in a minute, you're ready to attempt the 50-meter underwater swim.

You can learn about SFP super-burpees at:

www.SurvivalFitnessPlan.com/Daily-Conditioning-Workout/#Super_Burpees

Related Chapters:

- SFP Super-burpee
- Safety

MOUNTAIN BIKE RIDING

Most people know how to ride, but many do not know how to ride fast or through obstacles safely. This section will teach you how.

BASIC RIDING SKILLS

Braking

Use the brakes together. Pull the rear brake lever first, and then gradually squeeze the front as you brace yourself against the handlebars. Too much front brake, and you will go over the handle bars (endo); too much rear brake, and you will skid out of control.

The more weight over the wheel, the more stopping power it will have. Use this to your advantage. Leaning back while braking downhill will help to prevent endos, for example.

The faster you are going, the longer it will take to slow down. Keep your brakes covered at all times.

Using Gears

Higher gears are harder to pedal and will help you go faster. Lower gears are easier to pedal and help you get up hills. Shift before you get to the hill.

It is better to pedal faster in a low (easy) gear as opposed to slowly in a high gear.

Looking Ahead

As you ride, look ahead so you can adjust to any obstacles. Slow down for blind corners, and brake or steer early and smoothly rather than leaving it to the last minute.

BASIC DRILLS

Use the following drills to improve your basic riding skills.

Stand and Coast

Stand on your pedals without sitting on the seat and just coast. Keep your arms bent and don't lock your knees. Keep your pedals level.

Next, shift your body towards the rear of the bike. Use this position when coasting over obstacles or rough terrain.

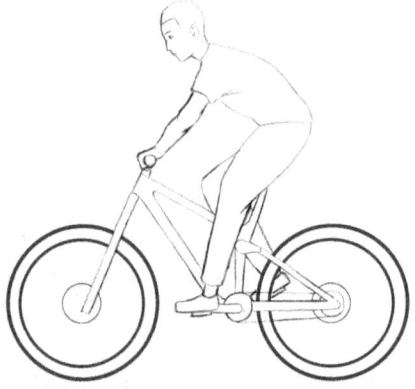

Stand and Pedal

Lift yourself off the seat and pedal.

Track Stand

Balance the bicycle in place, keeping your feet on the pedals. Use this technique when you have to move quickly, or to stop short to analyze an obstacle without losing your rhythm.

Coast at a slow speed, pedals level, and then come to a stop. Find your balance position. You can stand, sit, turn your wheel at an angle, etc.—whatever works for you.

Rock back and forth lightly. To rock forward, let off the brake a little. To rock back pull the bike back underneath you. Repeat this procedure.

Keep pressure on your front pedal while holding the brake to keep you in place.

Slow Ride

Ride between two points as slowly as possible without putting your foot down. Ride forward at all times—no zigzagging, etc.

Heel Grab

The goal is to grab onto one of your heels and keep riding along normally.

Pedal normally, then lean to your left and use your left hand to grab your left heel. Continue to hold your heel as you pedal. You can start off holding your calf, then move to your ankle, then your heel.

Bottle Pick Up

Ride towards an upright bottle so it is just off to your side. As you ride past the bottle, lean over and pick it up off the ground. Next, place it back on the ground in an upright position.

Slalom

Look straight ahead and weave in and out of a set of obstacles in a zigzag fashion—that is, to the left of the first obstacle, the right of the second, the left of the third etc. Start with the obstacles in a straight line about six feet apart and bring them closer together as you improve.

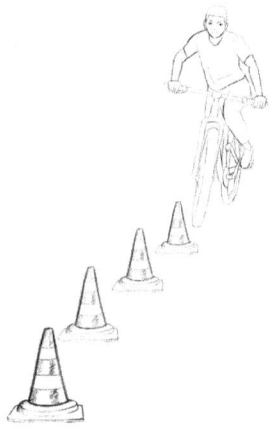

Offset Slalom

Use the same setup as with the regular slalom, but take every other cone and move it left or right by two or three feet. You'll have to take wider, sweeping turns and lean more to get around the obstacles. Continue to look ahead.

Figure 8's

Ride your bike in a figure eight in as small a space as possible without putting your foot down.

Gap Storming

Arrange two lines of cones in a V formation. Ride between them without hitting any. As your confidence increases, move the final pair closer and closer together.

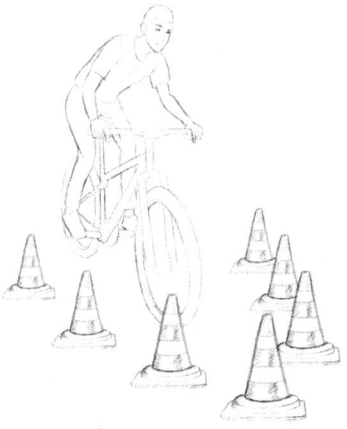

Down A Curb

Coast straight down off a curb. Absorb the drop with your arms and legs.

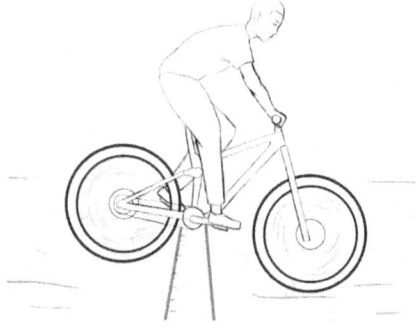

ADVANCED SKILLS

Fixing a Dropped Chain

If your chain drops onto the bottom bracket, just pedal easily and gently shift up with the big gears.

If the chain is jammed, get off the bike and manually put it back on.

If the chain falls outside the crank arm—on your foot, for example—then roll and shift down toward the small ring. You can use your foot to help place it back on.

Learning to Crash

Use the roll taught in parkour. Get comfortable doing a forward roll after a running dive. Progress the "crash" to rolling after slamming on your front brakes when riding on grass.

Cornering

Always look where you want to go. Anticipate the speed for the corner and brake before the corner if necessary. Never brake while turning. Approach the corner wide. Cut to the apex (the straightest line through a corner), and finish wide.

If you stop pedaling, put all your weight onto the outside pedal so it faces down towards the road. Resume peddling as soon as you have passed the apex.

Riding Faster

Push and pull the pedal around as if keeping the pedal to the outside of the circle. Lift your knees faster and higher.

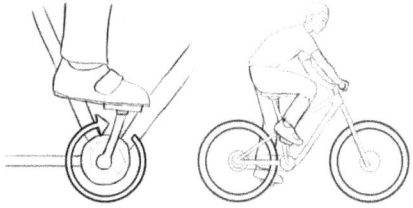

Uphill

If you need to shift during a climb, take a couple power strokes first. Soft pedal for a stroke while you shift, then pedal hard again.

On the road, you can stand, but on dirt, stay seated.

Slide your bum forward on your seat, and lean over the handlebars. Put your elbows back (not down). Pedal smoothly.

Downhill

To prevent the chain from falling off, shift into the big chain-ring.

Stand with pedals level and shift your weight over the back wheel. Stay loose on the bike. Don't lock your elbows or clench your grip. Steer with your body. Let your shoulders guide you.

Brake on solid dirt or rock where you can get traction, as opposed to on loose soil or gravel.

Floating Over Terrain

On rough terrain, let the bike float underneath you. It will move in different directions as it hits bumps. Keep your body upright and the bike pointed down the trail.

Looking Behind

Make sure the path ahead is clear. Relax your right arm to drop your shoulder a little. Your elbow should bend and your right hand should be relaxed. Turn your head left and slide your butt to the right as you glance over your shoulder.

Down A Ledge

Shift your weight back, drop your wrists to pull up the handlebars, and level the bike. Shift your weight forward as the rear wheel goes airborne.

Log Hopping

Get in the same position as if you were riding downhill.

Front Pull

Coast at medium speed and, without braking, push down on the handlebars. Pull upward and straighten your arms to bring the front wheel off the ground. Place it back down gently.

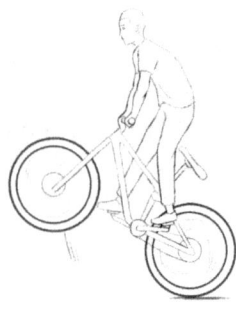

Hip-Hop

Shift your weight forward and turn your pedals so that your feet are almost vertical. Press back against the pedals as you push your legs up. Pull the back end up with your leg muscles, then bring it down gently.

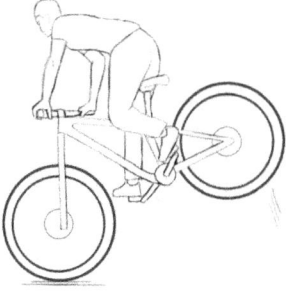

Log-Hopping

When you are log-hopping, the front pull and hip-hop become one motion. Perform the front pull and bring the wheel high enough to clear the log. Touch the front wheel on top of the log and, as the wheel starts to roll over it, do a hip-hop. If the log is wet, avoid touching your wheels on the top of it to prevent slipping.

Bunny-Hopping

A bunny-hop is similar to a log-hop, but with the intention of having both wheels off the ground at the same time.

Perform a front pull and while your front wheel is in the air, use the push/pull motion to get the back wheel up. Level your bike in the air and try to squeeze your legs together. Land your back wheel first.

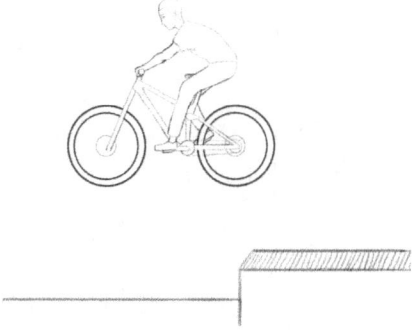

HIKING

To get the most benefit, go on long hikes and incorporate navigation training.

GENERAL HIKING TIPS

Find Your Pace

Your pace is how fast you walk. Develop a pace that you can maintain for a long time without requiring a break.

Take a series of five-minute walks while concentrating on maintaining pace length and speed. Find a pace that slightly raises your breathing but does not make you sweat.

Walk a known distance—from home to the corner store, for example—at this pace, and time how long it takes. Make the walk between 15 and 25 minutes. Repeat the same walk daily until you are covering the distance in a fairly consistent time. This is your steady pace.

Maintaining Your Pace

This is mental. Sing a song in rhythm with your steps, count your steps, breathe in time with your steps, etc.

Breathing

Use slow, deliberate, deep breaths from your stomach. On flat ground, use a three-to-three breathing rhythm. Inhale for three steps—right, left, right—and then exhale for three steps.

Taking Breaks

Apart from general rest, use breaks to stretch, refuel your body, go to the toilet, and identify/fix any potential problems with yourself or your gear.

Unless you're having a meal, keep your breaks short to prevent your muscles stiffening up.

Hiking with a Pack

Carry your pack with your legs. Fasten your hip belt snugly and adjust your shoulder straps so the bulk of the bag's weight rests on your hips.

Environment

Hiking is done in the elements. Watch out for dangerous plants and animals. Protect yourself from the sun. Don't freeze, overheat, or dehydrate.

SPECIFIC HIKING TIPS

Uphill

Refuel your body before ascending, and keep some snacks and water handy for during the climb.

Take smaller steps to maintain your pace. Avoid obstacles that require large steps.

On very steep ascents, zigzagging will reduce the gradient, but add distance.

Use a two-to-two breathing rhythm. That is, inhale for two steps and exhale for two steps.

If your pack straps are constricting you, loosen them.

Downhill

Keep your center of gravity over your legs. Don't lean forward or back. Stay light on your feet and keep your leg slightly bent as you plant it. Tightening your pack will improve your balance.

You may be tired from the ascent, but pay attention to your foot placement. If the decline is very steep, stand side-on and lower yourself down one step at a time. Zigzagging will help to slow your pace.

Off-Trail

Look for the path of least resistance. Check your bearings regularly. and do not rush. If possible, do not strap things to the outside of your pack.

Crossing Water

Triple-waterproof your gear. Take your hiking shoes and socks off and keep them dry.

Wider crossings usually bring shallower water, especially where ripples begin. Ripples also indicate rocks or faster flowing areas. Crossing downstream of larger rocks means less current and often an even floor.

Keep slow moving water below mid-thigh and fast-moving water below the knee. Plan where you will place each step. Face slightly upstream and slide your foot forward through the water.

Use a pole on the downstream side. Place it firmly, make sure it is stable, and lean on it as you step forward. Water that is deep and/or fast may pull at your poles.

If you are crossing with your pack on your back, undo your hip strap and remove one shoulder. If you're floating your pack across, have a tether as a back-up.

If you're swimming across, start upstream of your exit point. If you get swept downstream in rapids, float on your back with your feet downstream to absorb crashes. Use your hands to steer and work your way toward shore.

When you're in a group, put the strongest, biggest hiker on the upstream side.

Hot Weather

If possible, hike in forested land that follows a stream, or has stream crossings. Mountains are cooler than valleys.

Use electrolytes in your water, at half the strength of the recommended directions. Eat salty snacks while hiking.

Break more. Blisters will occur more readily.

Wear loose-fitting clothes. Polyester is better than cotton.

Cold Weather

Use the layer system. Use thermals. Avoid cotton. Cover/uncover your head to regulate heat.

Avoid sweating. If you start warming up, slow down. When you do sweat, take off layers and replace them during breaks.

Start your hike a little cold. If after 20 minutes of hiking you are still cold, add layers.

Use sunscreen and lip balm.

Eat small amounts often and continue to rehydrate. Tubes from hydration packs can freeze.

Hiking at Altitude

High-altitude hiking is trekking at an elevation that may affect your body. Some people are affected at as low as 7,000 feet.

Adjust your pace. Take deeper breaths and smaller steps. Perform two-to-two or one-to-one rhythmic breathing to adjust to the thinner air.

Use sunscreen and sunglasses. Weather can change quickly.

Desert Hiking

Don't count on finding water, even if there is some marked on your map.

Watch for distant storms and beware of flash floods.

Wear light clothes that cover your whole body. Use sunscreen, sunglasses, and insect repellent.

THANKS FOR READING

Dear reader,

Thank you for reading *Survival Fitness*.

If you enjoyed this book, please leave a review where you bought it. It helps more than most people think.

Don't forget your FREE book chapters!

You will also be among the first to know of FREE review copies, discount offers, bonus content, and more.

Go to:

https://offers.SFNonfictionBooks.com/Free-Chapters

Thanks again for your support.

REFERENCES

Back, J. (2011). *Horses, Hitches, and Rocky Trails: The Original Guide to Packing, Camping, and Getting Along with the Wilderness.* Skyhorse.

Canterbury D. (2014). *Bushcraft 101: A Field Guide to the Art of Wilderness Survival.* Adams Media.

Downs, T. Editors of Bicycling Magazine. (2010). *The Bicycling Guide to Complete Bicycle Maintenance & Repair: For Road & Mountain Bikes.* Rodale Books.

Fury, S. (2017). *Daily Health and Fitness.* SF Nonfiction Books.

Fury, S. (2017). *Emergency Roping and Bouldering.* SF Nonfiction Books.

Fury, S. (2017). *Essential Parkour Training.* SF Nonfiction Books.

Fury, S. (2018). *Survival Swimming.* SF Nonfiction Books.

HowExpert Press. (2011). *How To Mountain Bike: Your Step By Step Guide To Mountain Biking.* HowExpert.

Logue, V. (2004). *Hiking and Backpacking: Essential Skills, Equipment, and Safety.* Menasha Ridge Press.

Lopes, B. McCormack, L. (2010). *Mastering Mountain Bike Skills.* HowExpert.

Nealy, W. (1992). *Mountain Bike!: A Manual of Beginning to Advanced Technique.* Menasha Ridge Press.

AUTHOR RECOMMENDATIONS

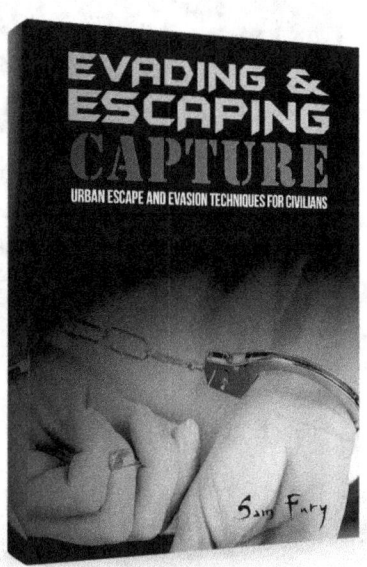

Teach Yourself Escape and Evasion Tactics

Discover the skills you need to evade and escape capture, because you never know when they will save your life.

Get it now.

www.SFNonfictionBooks.com/Evading-Escaping-Capture

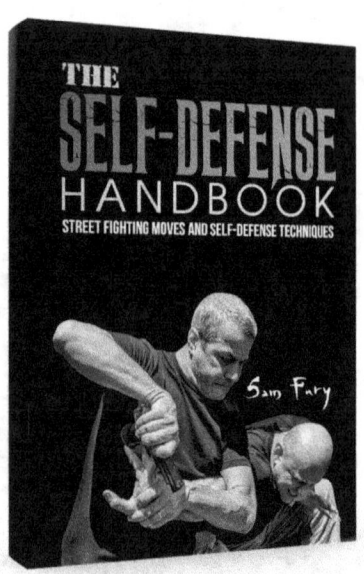

Teach Yourself Self-Defense

This is the only self-defense training manual you need, because these are the best street fighting moves around.

Get it now.

www.SFNonfictionBooks.com/Self-Defense-Handbook

ABOUT SAM FURY

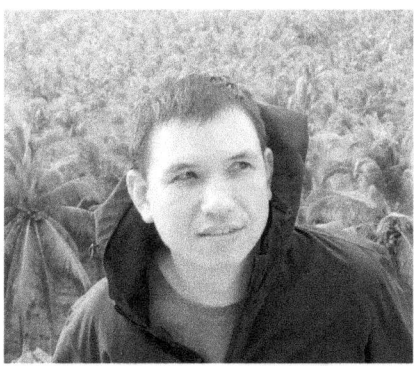

Sam Fury has had a passion for survival, evasion, resistance, and escape (SERE) training since he was a young boy growing up in Australia.

This led him to years of training and career experience in related subjects, including martial arts, military training, survival skills, outdoor sports, and sustainable living.

These days, Sam spends his time refining existing skills, gaining new skills, and sharing what he learns via the Survival Fitness Plan website.

www.SurvivalFitnessPlan.com

- amazon.com/author/samfury
- goodreads.com/SamFury
- facebook.com/AuthorSamFury
- instagram.com/AuthorSamFury
- youtube.com/SurvivalFitnessPlan

www.ingramcontent.com/pod-product-compliance
Lightning Source LLC
Chambersburg PA
CBHW071222080526
44587CB00013BA/1467